THE HORMONE BALANCE PLAN AND COOKBOOK

HOW A PLANT-BASED APPROACH CAN RESET YOUR ENDOCRINE SYSTEM, RESTORE ENERGY, & FIX YOUR METABOLISM

7 DAY MEAL PLAN WITH 21 DELICIOUS & SIMPLE RECIPES INCLUDED

Written By

PURETURE, HHP

PURETURE
HEALING THE FUTURE WITH PURE NATURE

CONTENTS

INTRODUCTION

"When diet is wrong, medicine is of no use. When diet is correct, medicine is of no need."

— ANCIENT AYURVEDIC PROVERB

Chronic health issues are a plague to our society. The CDC estimates that as many as 6 in 10 Americans suffer from one of many types of chronic health issues. (Centers for Disease Control, 2019) Of those 6 people, 4 of them will have more than one chronic health condition. Some of our most serious health concerns, including heart disease, diabetes, Alzheimer's disease, cancer, and endocrine disorders all fall under this massive umbrella of chronic health conditions.

You've picked up this book, so I'm guessing you're one of those 6 out of every 10, or you at least want to prevent yourself from becoming part of the statistics. Your health isn't what you want it to be, and you're tired of living each day feeling less like yourself and more like someone who is held down by pain, fatigue, mental fog, and a long list of other symptoms you don't want in your life. You're looking for a solution. Not a magic bullet that will fix your health temporarily by masking the symptoms, but true healing that will target the core issues that are affecting your health.

I'm someone who has lived through what you're experiencing. I've been living a clean, plant-based lifestyle for several years now, but it doesn't feel like that long ago that I was struggling with my health. I was experiencing hopelessness over whether I would ever have energy, feel those long-lost surges of vitality, or be able to avoid the mountain of prescription medications that were sure to come my way. I needed to take some sort of drastic measure to turn my health around.

I do want to say right now that the journey wasn't always easy. I had to dig deep and overcome the fears I had built up around my health. I also had to challenge what I thought about food and my emotional connection to it. I think we all want to feel more in control of our health but there's something about empowerment that can feel intimidating. Empowerment demands responsibility and a truthful acknowledgment of the challenges you're facing. This is not easy.

These years later, I can say I'm devoted to my plant-based lifestyle and I have helped clients improve their health by adopting many of the same dietary philosophies that I follow today. I know from my own experience and watching others that this type of change isn't just a physical one. It's also an emotional journey. We're talking about healthy changes that will sustain you throughout your entire life. True, sustainable healing of this type takes time and will affect you in ways you might have never imagined.

Adopting a plant-based lifestyle as much as possible at least, is beneficial in so many ways, including how it can help minimize disease and even prevent it. In this book, I've focused more specifically on hormonal health and autoimmune disease, particularly involving the endocrine system.

In the coming chapters, you're going to learn what an incredible and complex network the endocrine system is. You'll also learn more about the importance of hormonal balance in your overall health and wellbeing. The slightest imbalances in hormones can create a domino effect that may eventually lead to chronic disease, including autoimmune disorders.

If you're living with an autoimmune disorder, you already understand the challenging aspects of managing your disease. For the most part, there are no "cures" for autoimmune disease. Doctors focus mostly on relieving the most noticeable symptoms through medications, in hopes of slowing the progression of the disease. Unfortunately, many of these medications have serious side effects that are arguably as devastating as the disease itself.

When modern medicine isn't providing us with the answer we want, we have no choice but to turn back to ourselves for the solution. Many complementary therapies are effective in relieving the symptoms of chronic disease but none (at least in my opinion) are as crucial as diet when it comes to true healing. How we choose to nourish our bodies can influence not only whether disease develops but also whether or not we can heal from it.

Certain types of foods, such as meat, dairy, processed foods, and foods that are high in saturated fats and refined sugars are known to cause stress and harm to the body. This isn't just my opinion. There is evidence that has been revealed through years of ongoing research and studies on the effects of diet vs health. Plant-based foods have shown to be protective against the development of disease and also therapeutic, or even curative, against many types of chronic disease.

Here, we're going to look at the effects of adopting a plant-based diet on hormonal health, endocrine function, and autoimmune health. I want to share what I know through my professional experience, and what I have endured and experienced firsthand as I have worked to improve my own health and influence my personal outcomes for the future.

I know that adopting a plant-based lifestyle can help so many of you overcome the challenges of living with hormonal imbalance and autoimmune disorders. I know you have the power and are strong enough to make the changes. All you need is a foundation of knowledge in how it all works, proof that it's worth the effort, and some guidance on how to get started to achieve sustainable results.

RECOMMENDATION FROM THE PURETURE WELLNESS TEAM:

We would like to make this journey you are about to embark on as smooth as possible. As with any journey, preparations need to be made, and there are tools fit for each pilgrimage. In our case we require the Detox Goodies Toolkit, which is completely free. Not using these tools is like making a trip to a rainforest and not taking any sort of tool to protect yourself from mosquitoes. You can do it, but the experience won't be quite as seamless as it could have been. It is discomfort that is not necessary and can even be risky. This analogy fits perfectly; if you don't have the right tools to go through with this process it can be uncomfortable, and there is even a risk of failure involved.

Please access the following link: https://www.pureture.com/detox-goodies/

In this link you will find the following components:

- 20 Daily Detox Tips
- 15 Detox Tea Formulas
- 10 Detox Juices
- Master Shopping List: Healing & Detox Food

It may not be completely clear why these components are essential quite yet, but in further chapters you will notice that this information will be very helpful. When you actually begin the practical side of the work, you will come to understand. These tools are meant to alleviate some stress and obstacles that may show up along the way.

Are you ready to heal your hormones, reclaim your health, and refuse to fall victim to chronic disease that's influenced by dietary choices? Great, let's get started.

1

TAKING THE FIRST STEP

I f you're feeling less than your best these days, you're not alone. We're a society that's plagued by aches and pains, feeling "blah", and what sometimes seems like an endless list of chronic ailments. I've worked with enough clients over the years that I've been able to identify something that many of them have in common – their bodies are starving for nutrition and their hormones are unbalanced because of it.

I can sense that you might be raising an eyebrow at me right now. Neither hormones nor nutrition are common stopping points for treating chronic diseases and general unwellness. Many of us have never learned the important role that hormones play in our overall health or the lengthy list of diseases that can manifest when they're out of balance. We also haven't been taught how the right type of nourishment can restore that balance and rebuild health.

It isn't your fault that you haven't learned these things. Even medical doctors, whose very purpose it is to heal, lack formal education in the value of nutrition in healing the body. They're focused on providing a diagnosis and doing something to make you feel better, ASAP. When you go to the doctor, you want answers and relief. If a doctor told you to go home, eat a salad and call back in two weeks, you'd look at them like they were crazy.

We've been programmed to ignore the root cause and focus on immediate relief. This has fed into an ever-growing pharmaceutical industry that doesn't always have your best interest in mind. Don't get me wrong, modern medicine, including pharmaceuticals, are valuable. The problem is we turn to medications too often to relieve symptoms without taking the time to address what's causing the disharmony in the first place. You get relief but you never get better.

There are countless causes of disease – more than we could ever properly discuss in one book. Each person's body also responds differently to various factors that can contribute to disease or dis-ease. We all know that person who seems to dodge every bullet when it comes to disease, yet also know someone else who seems to attract disease and disharmony like a magnet. There aren't always easy explanations for these scenarios.

There is one cause of disease that isn't talked about enough – hormones. That weight gain that seemed to come out of

nowhere? Probably hormones. Diabetes? hormones. Sleepless-
ness, irritability, skin issues? Yes, hormones. Thyroid disease,
PCOS, metabolic syndrome? All because of hormones.

If there's one thing the traditional medical community is lacking, it is an effective way of addressing hormone-related conditions without automatically prescribing a medication. I want to
say here that for some hormone-related diseases, you should
absolutely trust your doctor in prescribing medications. Sometimes, these diseases can be life-threatening, and medication can
help reduce the immediate risk.

That said, medications don't work for all hormone imbalances,
and nutrition is an often-overlooked therapy. Depending on the
hormone imbalance you suffer from, nutritional therapy
through plant-based eating and structured detox can be the only
treatment you need.

I feel very strongly that knowledge is power, no matter what
situation you're facing. We're going to get our feet wet here by
learning more about the role hormones play in your overall
health, and about a very important part of your body called the
endocrine system.

How and Why the Endocrine System Is So Important to Your Health

The endocrine system is somewhat of an unsung hero. The
endocrine system is responsible for controlling and regulating

an incredible range of functions, many of which go unnoticed until symptoms of imbalance begin to manifest. The endocrine system controls several physiological functions through the release of hormones that make their way through your body, eventually reaching organs and tissues where they perform vital work.

The whole of the endocrine system is a network of glands, that when functioning properly, produce and secrete hormones. When we start talking about hormones, we immediately think about the role they play in key transitional life phases, like adolescence, pregnancy, and menopause. What many people don't know is that hormones play a hugely important role in health, outside of their roles that we're more familiar with.

Hormones are chemical substances. As the glands of your endocrine system release hormones, they set off to targeted destinations within the body where they regulate all sorts of cellular and organ activity. In youth, hormones regulate growth, which includes a whole myriad of body systems – skeletal, muscular, reproductive, cardiovascular, etc. As we mature, hormones take on many roles, and when an imbalance occurs, we see it manifested in many of the chronic diseases we see today.

A few of the primary jobs of the endocrine system include:

- Regulating growth and development during youth, adolescence, and young adulthood

- Sexual reproduction
- Regulating metabolism so that your body doesn't metabolize energy too fast or too slow
- Maintaining the delicate balance of your internal body systems – a process called homeostasis
- Controlling your response to stimuli, including how you react to fear, stress, fatigue, injury, etc.

This list looks pretty simple but in reality, each is complex. To illustrate, think about what we know about the long-term effects of chronic stress. It all starts with how the endocrine system responds and functions to restore a state of balance. An endocrine system that works too hard, or not hard enough, in response to stimuli is going to cause havoc in your body.

Soon, we'll dig deeper and talk about endocrine disorders and how they're affecting our health on such a wide scale. Before we do that, I want to take a step back and talk about the different glands that make up the endocrine system, and the important role that each one plays.

The glands of the endocrine system include:

Hypothalamus – The hypothalamus is a small gland, about the size of an almond, located in the brain. This small gland carries the heavy responsibility of helping your body sustain homeostasis and keeping many functions of the autonomous nervous system in check.

The hypothalamus is responsible for regulating body temperature, thirst, appetite, weight gain, heart rate, sleep, and blood pressure. It also partners with and supports the pituitary gland. Who says big things don't come in small packages?

Pituitary Gland – The pituitary gland is located right below the hypothalamus at the base of the brain. Being only about the size of a pea, this tiny powerhouse consists of two lobes that produce hormones that send signals to the other glands of the endocrine system. The pituitary gland produces growth hormone, thyroid-stimulating hormone, prolactin, and other hormones that influence reproduction.

Thyroid – The thyroid gland's key responsibility is to produce two hormones that we call T3 and T4 (triiodothyronine and thyroxine if you want to be more technical). These hormones are metabolism regulators. They help your body break down food for energy and utilize it. Even slight disturbances in T3 or T4 production can have a noticeable impact on weight loss or weight gain. However, to say that weight control and metabolism are the extents of the thyroid's duties is an understatement. The thyroid, and the hormones it produces, are involved in many crucial processes.

Parathyroid – We don't hear a whole lot about these little grain-sized glands. As the name suggests, they're located close to the thyroid gland, but they work completely independently. There are four parathyroid glands, and they work together to regulate body calcium levels. Calcium is important for muscular and skeletal health, but calcium also plays a crucial role in the nervous and cardiovascular system.

Adrenal Gland – You have two adrenal glands that sit just above your kidneys. Each adrenal gland contains two parts – the adrenal cortex and the adrenal medulla. The function of the adrenals that most people are aware of is the production of adrenaline – a hormone released in response to stimuli that produces a fight or flight response and causes a surge in energy. Your adrenals also produce the stress hormone cortisol and its inflammation regulating partner corticosterone.

Pineal Gland – The pineal gland is located deep within the center of the brain, which helps to explain why of all the glands in the endocrine system, this is the one that was discovered last. Unlike the other multi-tasking glands of the endocrine system, the pineal gland has one primary purpose – to produce the hormone melatonin.

You might recognize melatonin as the sleep-aid found in the vitamin and supplement aisle. Melatonin regulates your body's circadian rhythm. When working properly, levels of melatonin are lower during the day and higher in the evening as bedtime nears. Melatonin also plays an important role in reproductive functions.

Thymus – The thymus gland is arguably the most peculiar of the endocrine system. This gland which is located between your lungs doesn't function throughout your entire life. As you age it disappears entirely to be replaced by fatty tissue.

The thymus is active only in childhood and starts to wind-down its work once a person reaches puberty. The thymus is crucial in the development of the immune system. It produces thymosin, a hormone that promotes the development of T-cells, which are your body's disease-fighting warriors.

Ovaries/Testes – Most people are familiar with ovaries and testes as reproductive glands. The ovaries in females secrete estrogen and progesterone, while the testes in men secrete testosterone. These glands and hormones are essential to reproductive development in adolescence and support reproductive health into adulthood. As we age, the levels of hormones produced by the ovaries and testes begin to naturally decline.

Pancreas – Yes, the pancreas is an organ, but it is made of two separate parts that function as glands – the endocrine pancreas and the exocrine pancreas. The endocrine pancreas secretes the hormones insulin and glucagon, which work to regulate blood glucose levels. The exocrine pancreas plays a key role in digestive processes.

When thinking about your overall health and wellbeing, it's important to see all the different working parts and systems of your body as all being interconnected. When all is in balance, each system works beautifully. When something is out of whack, it can create a domino effect with far-reaching effects on your health. This is especially true for the endocrine system, which works hand in hand with your nervous, digestive, and cardiovascular systems.

The endocrine system is also supported by other organs in the body. Vital organs, such as the heart, kidneys, and liver all perform what we call secondary endocrine functions. This means that in addition to their primary function, they also produce and secrete hormones. For example, we're all familiar with the importance and main purpose of the heart but it also performs secondary endocrine functions. When the heart is under pressure from increased blood volume, it produces a hormone called an atrial natriuretic peptide, or ANP for those of you who don't like tongue twisters. This hormone works with the kidneys to reduce blood volume and pressure, saving you from a catastrophic cardiovascular event.

The endocrine system is so intertwined with every organ and tissue in your body that it's impossible to not see how imbalances in any gland or hormone production can affect your overall state of health and well-being. Endocrine disorders are an ever-growing health challenge, especially in the United States.

What Is an Endocrine Disorder?

The human body is an amazing machine, but we all know that it isn't infallible. We all experience things, sometimes daily, that reinforce this unfortunate truth. Whether it's coming down with a cold, nursing a sprained ankle, suffering through a migraine, or coping with a chronic disease, many things can throw the body off balance.

An unhealthy, out of balance endocrine system can lead to any number of diseases that we call endocrine disorders. It's almost mind-boggling when you start looking at the number of diseases that are caused by hormonal imbalance and endocrine dysfunction. We'll cover specific endocrine disorders in more detail in this chapter, but endocrine disorders are behind some of the most serious, chronic diseases we're facing today.

A serious problem that exists for many people with an endocrine disorder is that they're either misdiagnosed or self-diagnosed, which prevents the person from being able to work towards balance and healing. As we go deeper into our discussion about hormonal health and how diet plays a crucial role, it's important to remember that the first discussion you need to have is with your medical care provider.

If you're interested in treating your endocrine disorder or hormonal imbalance holistically and naturally, find a health care provider/practitioner who is aligned with your views on how to approach your health. It frustrates me when I see people doing a sort of battle with their healthcare providers because they are on completely different pages. However, working with someone who can diagnose and help set you on the path to wellbeing is essential. There is a tremendous amount of work that you can do to take back control of your hormonal health, but this isn't a journey that you should travel completely alone.

Why Are Endocrine Disorders So Prevalent Today?

When talking on this topic, I'm often asked how prevalent endocrine disorders are today. This is a difficult question to answer and it's because the reach of these types of disorders goes so very deep into our society. For starters, endocrine disorders are extremely prevalent, especially in the western world. Exact numbers of people who are affected by them are hard to come by for a few different reasons.

Studies have attempted to measure the prevalence of endocrine disorders as a whole within our society. The difficulty comes with the fact that there are so many different endocrine disorders, and they often go undiagnosed for years until the disease progresses to the point that it begins to manifest more serious, noticeable symptoms.

Another issue is that endocrine disorders often overlap. For example, obesity and diabetes are both considered endocrine disorders. They also often present as comorbid conditions. It's not uncommon for a singular person to be coping with more than one endocrine-related disorder. This makes tracking these conditions and putting their numbers into nice little compartments even more challenging.

I mentioned that endocrine disorders are a serious health issue here in the western world, but they also affect a huge portion of the global population. It's interesting to look at which endocrine disorders are most prevalent in different parts of the world and compare that data to possible causes.

According to the European Society of Endocrinology, thyroid disease is one of the most common endocrine disorders in Europe. (Elisei & Alvarez) In the United States, diabetes is the most commonly diagnosed endocrine disorder. While type 1 diabetes is genetically influenced, type 2 is far more common and almost always influenced by dietary factors. Interestingly, two different areas of the world face different challenges with endocrine disease. We're all of the same species, so why such different statistics?

Honestly, the whole answer to this is a much more complex puzzle than we can unfold here in this book. However, dietary influences are a huge factor in the development and aggressiveness of endocrine disorders. On the flip side, dietary changes can also be one of your strongest paths back toward health.

To understand why endocrine disorders are so prevalent today, let's start by looking at what the nutritional community refers to as the Standard American Diet, or it's aptly named acronym, SAD. The SAD diet is characterized by a significant intake of animal protein, especially red meat, and processed meats, as well as other animal products, high-fat dairy, refined sugars, fried foods, processed foods, and refined grains. The typical SAD diet is also rather limited in the intake of nutrient-dense fruits, vegetables, and whole grains.

The problem with the SAD diet is that it doesn't support your health in any way. It lacks nutrients and is high in fats, sugars, and artificial ingredients. When you consume the typical SAD diet, you might be filling your body, but you aren't nourishing it. Your body has to work overtime to process everything you consume, and it's doing so with minimal nutritional support. Inflammation, hormonal imbalance, and chronic health issues are the body's natural response to essentially starving from nutrition and healing it has needed for years.

In the United States, it's estimated that three-fourths of the population consumes a diet that is low in vegetables, fruits, and oils. (U.S. Department of Health and Human Services). When I say oil, I'm not referring to fat – we're getting plenty of that. I'm referring to vegetable-based oils, like olive oil or avocado oil, that are thought to have some redeemable healthy qualities.

The natural consequence of the SAD is weight gain, but it seems like we all know that one person that has an "incredible" metabolism and can eat whatever they want and not gain an ounce. In my experience, it's safe to say that even people who appear to outwardly suffer no consequences of the SAD way of eating do face endocrine-related health challenges that can be connected directly back to their diet.

If you're someone who has grown up eating SAD, or as an adult have struggled with the willpower or even desire to change your eating patterns, know that I'm not saying any of this to shame you. We develop such a powerful connection with food, and many of us tend to take any criticism of our dietary habits very personally.

What I am hoping to do here is inform those who are struggling with hormone imbalance, and any related health condition, that the prevalence of endocrine disorders is, in a large part, our own doing.

As a society, we've spent decades turning to foods that offered convenience and immediate satiation, as opposed to choosing foods that truly nourish our bodies. This has resulted in the epidemic of endocrine disorders we're seeing today. There's good news here, too. You have it completely within your power to turn away from one of the leading causes of endocrine disorders and reshape your future health.

Who Suffers from Endocrine Disorders?

Many people don't realize how commonly diagnosed endocrine disorders are. Once you begin to learn some of the diseases that fall under the umbrella of an endocrine disorder, this point of view instantly changes. So many of the most common chronic health conditions that we see today are directly related to hormonal imbalance and ineffective endocrine function.

Something else that I've noticed is that there is a common misconception about who suffers from endocrine disorders. Mention the word "hormone" concerning a health condition and many will just assume that you're talking about women's health. Women indeed go through several important hormonal phases throughout their lives, and as a result, can have a predisposition to hormonal imbalance. However, endocrine disorders do not affect just women. Men also suffer in great numbers, especially from endocrine-related conditions like obesity, diabetes, and low testosterone.

With many diseases, age is a significant contributing factor. Some diseases tend to affect younger people – like testicular cancer in men, while others like heart disease increase in prevalence as we age. Endocrine disorders are different in this regard.

Hormones are important to your health throughout your entire life. Your body is always producing hormones, and natural levels tend to shift over time. Because the importance of hormones spans your entire life, so does the potential for endocrine dysfunction.

Endocrine disorders can affect children and adolescents in ways that you might see delayed growth and maturation, or the opposite end of the spectrum with precocious puberty. Thyroid cancer tends to affect younger adults, with an average age range of diagnosis being between 20-45 years, with the peak incidence occurring toward the latter end of that spectrum. (NCRAS)

Infertility affects both men and women in their main reproductive years, obesity and diabetes don't discriminate based on age, and older adults are more susceptible to endocrine-related health issues like heart disease and osteoporosis. The point is that endocrine health is important no matter your age and taking steps to heal and protect it should be a top priority, regardless if you are 22 or 82.

I've just mentioned a few of the different endocrine disorders but there are so many more. The sheer number of endocrine disorders is a little overwhelming, especially if this is your first step to healing and protecting your hormonal health. One source lists 48 different endocrine diseases. Of course, some of these are rare, but others serve as more of an umbrella category. For example, "reproduction" is listed as an endocrine disorder, which can easily splinter off into many different individual reproduction-related conditions.

In the next chapter, we're going to talk about some of the most common endocrine disorders, along with a few of the less common ones. I'm also going to list some signs and symptoms of your endocrine system being out of whack. If you find that your health issues match up with those symptoms, I urge you to discuss your concerns with a health practitioner, even if you don't think you have one of the more common conditions that we're going to talk about here.

I've worked directly with people who just didn't feel "right", and it wasn't until after an actual diagnosis and taking charge of their health that they realized how significant their symptoms were. Just because you don't see yourself in one of the endocrine disorders we're going to talk about here, doesn't mean that endocrine dysfunction isn't a problem for you.

Treating Endocrine Disorders

Endocrine disorders are so different and complex. There isn't a single treatment or remedy that the traditional medical community can supply that will treat each disorder effectively. Add to this the different factors that contribute to any individual's endocrine dysfunction, and you've got a situation that is nothing short of a medical puzzle that needs to be slowly unraveled before it can be solved.

I'm not here to discredit the value of traditional medicine, especially when it comes to the diagnosis of endocrine disorders and the treatment of serious diseases, such as endocrine cancers. What I have found in my work is that many people who have been diagnosed with an endocrine disorder are, at best, frustrated with the traditional courses of treatment prescribed by medical doctors.

In most cases, a doctor is going to first prescribe pharmaceuticals that control the symptoms of the endocrine disorder before they even begin to think about addressing the root cause. They might tell a patient to lose weight, increase physical activity, or reduce stress along with taking their medication but the patient is often left up to their own devices in learning how to make those changes.

I believe that you can't approach disease treatment without first looking at the root cause and addressing how to treat the core of the problem, rather than just the symptoms. Considering the role that dietary and lifestyle choices play in the development of endocrine disorders, this is one of the first places we should look when it comes to uncovering and healing the root cause.

I once worked with a client that was suffering from severe hormonal irregularities that were associated with menopause. She was dealing with extreme hot flashes – the type that kept her up all night and interfered with her ability to focus and function during the day. The thing is, menopause is a natural, hormonal transition for women, so the medical community tends to see all the discomforts and physical stress of menopause as something that is just a fact of this stage of life for women. Their only solution is to offer hormonal replacements that work to synthetically balance hormonal levels.

Hormone therapy isn't right for everyone. It's contraindicated for women with certain health conditions. In this case, the client I was working with was not interested in synthetic hormones to control her menopausal symptoms. She wanted her body to be in balance, and she knew that it could be achieved naturally with a little guidance.

For this client, I took the approach of specifically designing a detox program that would help balance her hormones and ease her symptoms and discomfort as her body navigated this transition. After completing the detox, she claimed her hot flashes were completely gone. This is a perfect example of how treating the root cause by bringing the body back into balance and harmony naturally can treat endocrine disorders.

Of course, the main premise of this book is how choosing a plant-based diet over the typical SAD way of eating can reverse the processes that are causing hormonal imbalance. Take, for instance, autoimmune disorders. An autoimmune disorder is when the body basically produces a super immune response and attacks itself. This creates excessive, chronic inflammation.

Autoimmune diseases, like rheumatoid arthritis, Crohn's disease, and lupus create systemic inflammation. When this type of inflammation is present, your body is experiencing a great deal of stress. It responds by putting the endocrine system into action, which under normal circumstances isn't a bad thing. But when stress is chronic, the continual activation of the endocrine system and release of hormones results in imbalances, which only add to the fuel for the autoimmune disease. It's a terrible cycle that often continues unbroken.

I've found that, for people with an autoimmune disease, treating hormonal imbalances through a plant-based diet can have a therapeutic effect on the root of the autoimmune disease itself. This isn't just me loving plants and wanting to share my enthusiasm with everyone. There's science that also backs up the theory that plant-based eating is effective in treating or at least minimizing the severity of certain autoimmune diseases. (Alwarith, Kahleova, Rembert, Yonas, Dort, Calcagno., . . . Barnard, 2019)

The Next Step

Now that we've built a foundation of understanding endocrine disorders, it's time to start looking forward to the next step – learning how and why plant-based nutrition is key to achieving a healthy, balanced body.

CHAPTER SUMMARY

In this chapter, we've learned about the endocrine system – what it is, the glands involved, and a brief introduction to how each affects your health. We've also had an introduction to endocrine disorders and why they're so prevalent today. Specifically, we've discussed:

- How nutrition and hormone regulation go hand in hand, yet nutrition is an often-overlooked remedy in treating endocrine disorder;
- How the endocrine system is a network of glands that control physiological functions through the release of hormones;

- How endocrine health is important throughout your life, from infancy on;
- How endocrine disorders are commonly misdiagnosed, leading to infective treatment;
- How nutrition and incorporating more plant-based foods into your diet is one of the most effective treatments and preventative measures against endocrine disorders.

In the next chapter, we're going to take a closer look at specific endocrine disorders, what causes them, and the best plant-based foods to help balance hormones and heal your endocrine system.

2

THE KEY TO A BALANCED BODY IS A BALANCED DIET

Now that you've become a little more familiar with the endocrine system, you can see how the different glands affect the entire body. Hormonal health is important no matter what stage of life you're currently in or preparing for.

There are plenty of arguments that can be made for instilling healthy eating habits in our children. One of the most important is that by teaching our children to make choices that nourish their bodies, we're setting them up for a lifetime of hormonal well-being. Young bodies are very much influenced by endocrine health and the sooner we provide dietary support to the endocrine system, the better.

In this chapter, we're going to talk about why it's important to adopt healthy dietary habits now, more specifically, why you should be looking more towards plant-based nutrition to support endocrine health. We're also going to take a closer look at the more specific ways endocrine dysfunction affects your long-term health.

What Types of Endocrine Disorders Are There?

When we start looking at the number of endocrine disorders, we realize there is so much here to uncover. As of now, there are at least four dozen recognized endocrine disorders, although many of them are considered rare. The scientific community is always working to understand more about the endocrine system and its connection to disease. As we learn, we discover a deeper relationship between endocrine function and many of the chronic illnesses people are suffering from today.

In the United States, diabetes, a disease that involves the pancreas and the production of insulin, is hands down the most commonly diagnosed endocrine disorder. Fortunately, it's also one that is most receptive to healing through plant-based eating.

While diabetes is the most common endocrine disorder, it's far from being the only one we need to be focusing on. Other common endocrine disorders include:

- *Hyperthyroidism* – An endocrine disease characterized by the overproduction of thyroid hormones.
- *Hypothyroidism* – The opposite of hyperthyroidism,

this occurs when the thyroid under produces thyroid hormones.

- *Polycystic ovary syndrome (PCOS)* – This occurs when the androgen hormones are overproduced and interfere with the development and release of mature egg cells from the ovaries.
- *Precocious puberty* – A endocrine disorder that has been on the rise during recent years, precocious puberty occurs when a child, male or female, enters puberty before the typical age of onset.
- *Cushing's Disease* – Caused by the overproduction of hormones within the pituitary gland, leading to excessive adrenal involvement
- *Adrenal insufficiency* – This occurs when the adrenal glands underproduce the hormones cortisol and aldosterone.
- *Low testosterone* – Caused by an underproduction of testosterone in the sex glands.
- *Osteoporosis* – A disease of a porous bone structure where the quality and density of bone material is degraded. We don't think of osteoporosis as having anything to do with hormones, however, the role of the parathyroid in calcium synthesis can greatly influence the development of this disease.
- *Leaky gut* – Leaky gut is a condition that involves higher than normal gut permeability. A healthy gut works off a delicate balance. In the case of leaky gut,

the gut biome has deteriorated, making it possible for bacteria and toxins to permeate the gut lining. It's thought that stress and hormonal imbalance are contributing factors to leaky gut syndrome.

There's one more endocrine-related that I want to talk about here, but I feel like it needs a little more explanation. In the above list, I briefly touched on adrenal insufficiency. There's another related condition called adrenal fatigue that I'd like to talk about in a little more detail.

First, I want to start by saying that adrenal fatigue isn't a recognized medical term. If you were to mention this to a medical doctor, the range of responses might be anything from acknowledgment to an eye-roll. Adrenal fatigue is a term used to describe a grouping of non-specific symptoms that can all be tied back to insufficient adrenal function. The problem is that while there are tests to measure adrenal insufficiency, the current blood tests aren't sensitive enough to pick up on the slightest fluctuations in adrenal function that can have non-specific effects on your health.

The idea behind adrenal fatigue is that the adrenal glands simply can't keep up with the stress we're putting them through every day. Our current lifestyle, where we're always on the go, pushing ourselves to the limit every day, and taking on stress from things happening in the world around us keeps us in a perpetual fight or flight mode. This is certain to put stress on your adrenal glands, to the point that they cease to function optimally, even if the actual difference can't be detected by a simple blood test.

The symptoms of adrenal fatigue can be quite general and include body aches that come and go, general fatigue, dizziness, mood changes, unexplained weight loss, and changes to normal blood pressure.

Symptoms of Endocrine Disorders

My clients are often curious about the symptoms of endocrine disorders. This is such a difficult question to answer because unlike other types of diseases, endocrine disorders are each so different. The symptoms of endocrine disorders are different depending on the disease and how the person's body is responding to it.

Still, we're curious creatures that want some sort of answer. The best we can do here is provide a list of symptoms that are associated with some of the most common endocrine disorders, such as diabetes and adrenal insufficiency. The list of possible symptoms includes:

- Fatigue
- Excessive thirst
- Weight loss or gain
- Vision changes
- Changes in appetite

- Headache
- Nausea
- Menstrual irregularities
- Hair loss
- Skin discolorations
- Depression
- Anxiety

The Many Causes of Endocrine Disorders

My main focus is to provide you with information about how adopting a plant-based lifestyle can positively affect your health, specifically concerning hormonal health. It goes without saying that diet itself can lead to endocrine disruption but that isn't the only cause. It's equally important to recognize the other causes of endocrine disorders so we can better understand healing and how adopting a plant-based lifestyle can influence health outcomes.

Here are a few of the most common causes behind endocrine disorders, outside of lifestyle and dietary factors. Keep in mind that this list isn't exhaustive. The endocrine system is complex and can be affected by any number of factors.

Endocrine Disrupting Chemicals (EDCs)

Endocrine-disrupting chemicals (EDGs) come from environmental sources. They're substances we come in contact with daily that can negatively affect endocrine function. EDCs are difficult to avoid because they're found practically everywhere. They're in the soil, the air we breathe, and even in our water supplies.

We also get plenty of exposure to EDCs through personal care products and certain foods. A few examples of EDCs include:

- Industrial chemicals that make their way into the air
- Pesticides that leach into soil and groundwater. This is a risk even if you're consuming pesticide-free foods because these chemicals can reach animals who may eventually contribute to the food chain
- Non-organic fruits and vegetables that contain pesticide residues. This can come from spraying the produce or, in some cases, through absorption from the water and soil
- Processed foods that come in contact with EDCs through the manufacturing and production process
- Materials such as flooring and furniture, particularly those that are flame retardant
- Household and personal care products that can leach EDCs from their containers. Fragranced items, such as

lotions and creams, and household cleansers are major culprits

You might remember back in 2012, when after several states had taken a stand against BPA, the FDA banned the chemical in certain products, more specifically baby bottles, and sippy cups. The reason for this is, after a long history of concerns being raised, it was finally determined that the BPA in baby bottles and sippy cups could leach into the food and drink they contained, posing a risk to endocrine development in small children. Many companies followed suit, committing to providing BPA free packaging (Houlihan, Lunder, & Jacob).

BPA is just one example of an EDC you may be familiar with. As for BPA-free bottles, cups, dishes, etc., keep in mind that BPA isn't the only EDC that is found in materials such as plastic. BPA-free is a good start, but choosing glass, stainless steel (food grade), or bamboo is a much safer option.

Genetic Risk

Sometimes a person's predisposition to endocrine dysfunction has little to do with their lifestyle habits or external influences. Genetics can also play a critical role in how endocrine dysfunction manifests itself. From the point of conception, our genetic makeup is already in place. Genetic mutations occur quite frequently, many of them we never even know about. However, some mutations can have noticeable or serious effects on a person's health.

The thing about genetic predisposition is that you can't outgrow a genetic disorder, and it simply doesn't vanish one day. These are conditions that a person must learn to live with, and in some cases, adapt their lives to best cope with the effects.

Diabetes is an interesting example of the difference between lifestyle vs genetic risk in the development of endocrine disease. According to the CDC, more than 1 million adults in the United States are living with diabetes or prediabetes. (Centers for Disease Control and Prevention. 2017) Type II diabetes, which is the most common, is caused primarily by dietary and lifestyle factors, although age typically plays a role as well. On the other hand, type I diabetes is purely genetic, and tends to present itself much earlier in life, often during childhood or young adulthood.

Diabetes is a disease that affects how the body produces and utilizes the hormone insulin. Because of the genetic component, people with type I diabetes often have a more serious disease and have a more difficult time managing their symptoms.

Genetics can influence a person's risk of other endocrine disorders, such as thyroid cancer, sex chromosome abnormalities, polycystic ovarian syndrome, and some metabolic conditions.

However, adopting a healthier diet and lifestyle will contribute to keeping any unwanted symptoms at bay and make them much more manageable than you would likely experience when eating foods that aren't the most beneficial for these predispositions.

Autoimmune Disorders

When you stop to think about everything your immune system does daily, it's truly remarkable. Your immune system protects you from all sorts of pathogens and works tirelessly to keep you healthy. Most of us are familiar with how it feels when our immune system isn't up to par. Things like stress or lack of sleep can break down the immune system to the point that it doesn't protect us as well as it normally does.

There's another side to this coin, and it's when the immune system works "too" well. Instead of recognizing and launching an attack against bacteria, viruses, and other foreign invaders, the immune system turns on itself, unable to differentiate between parts of the body and pathogens. This is a simplistic explanation of autoimmune disorders, but you can see how this creates a scenario where the immune system is always on, supercharged, and constantly attacking healthy cells, tissues, and organs.

Currently, we know of at least 100 different autoimmune diseases, each affecting the body differently. While autoimmune disease is sometimes confined to a specific part of the body, for instance, the digestive tract in Crohn's disease or the skin in psoriasis, these conditions are almost always systemic. They produce a string of related symptoms that affect the body as a whole. One common symptom of autoimmune disease is systemic inflammation.

This is where we start getting into how autoimmune disease is related to endocrine function. We know that inflammation increases cortisol production, which puts additional stress on the endocrine system. We also see sex hormones come into play with certain autoimmune disorders, like Graves' disease and Hashimoto's thyroiditis, being more prominent in women. Autoimmune diseases can create this sort of catch-22 situation where the disease develops, at least in part, due to hormonal imbalance. Then the cycle of disease puts greater stress on the endocrine system, sometimes leading to more serious endocrine disorders.

Medications and Supplements

Any medication, drug, or supplement that disrupts hormonal balance can lead to the development of an endocrine disorder. There are some medications and supplements that are obvious endocrine disruptors – think along the line of hormonal contraceptives or supplements used to ease the symptoms of menopause. Many times, these types of medications are important in a person's life, and depending on the circumstance, the potential risk to endocrine balance is far outweighed by the benefit received.

Still, it's important to understand that medications and supplements that interfere with natural hormone production carry the potential to be disruptive to endocrine function. There are also other types of medications that are known endocrine disruptors that aren't as obvious.

For example, benzodiazepines can stress adrenal and pituitary function. Opioids and steroids can interfere with sex hormone production. If you're taking any medication, it's always wise to have a discussion with your healthcare provider regarding the range of potential side effects, including endocrine disruption.

It might not be advised that you cease taking medication based on these side effects, but you will be armed with the knowledge that you need to take extra steps to protect endocrine balance while taking them. It can also be recommended that you discuss with your doctor about designing a plan that can help you in the direction of achieving your goals without the use of medication for long periods of time.

Infection and Traumatic Injury

Occasionally, infection and traumatic injury, including surgery, can lead to endocrine imbalance. Any infection that affects hormone production or synthesis, or an event that produces a long-term inflammatory response, puts you at a greater risk of developing endocrine-related health conditions.

How a Plant-Based Diet Positively Affects Hormones

So, now we get to the part that I'm really excited to share with you. Helping people achieve optimal health through holistic means is a true passion of mine. To me, the idea that plants – the very bounty supplied by mother nature – are capable of healing our bodies, is incredible. The beauty of whole, nutritious foods, particularly plants, is that they nourish the body, providing everything that it needs to heal and perform optimally, without containing anything that inhibits natural hormonal function. It's a true lightbulb moment when you realize that focusing more on plant-based eating is the way things should have been all along.

I've said it previously, but I feel it deserves repeating. We build such emotional connections to our food. We build memories around food, associate them with our culture and upbringing. Food is incredibly personal. For many people, adopting a plant-based lifestyle disrupts the emotional connection they have with food, and not always in a good way. There are some of you out there who will be very resistant to making a full-throttle leap towards plant-based living. I want you to know that while seeing you embrace the lifestyle completely would thrill me, I understand that baby steps are easier, and more achievable.

I'd go as far as to say that you don't have to adopt a completely plant-based lifestyle but rather make it the center of your diet. If you can do this and cut out refined and processed foods, then you've made a huge first step toward reclaiming your health.

All that said, I think by the time you finish this book, you'll no longer view dietary changes as challenges but something that you whole-heartedly embrace. You're here because you don't like how you feel, your health isn't what it once was, and you're tired of feeling bullied by your body. You want to take back the control, and I want to help you do it.

The first way that plant-based eating supports your hormone health is that it doesn't place unnecessary stress on your body. When you ingest foods that are highly processed or loaded with fats and sugar, your body almost immediately begins to respond. It has to work harder and work longer to extract any nutrients and then process and release toxins. In contrast, whole foods, including plants, produce the opposite effect.

Your diet can also affect specific hormones individually. For example, cortisol levels increase when you consume refined sugars and other foods that are high on the GI scale. Whole, plant-based foods can lower cortisol levels, reduce systemic stress, and provide nutrients that support both physical and mental health. Foods rich in magnesium, like spinach and legumes, also help keep hormone levels in check.

Whole foods are also associated with a better metabolic response. They support healthy metabolic rates and long-term weight management. Weight management isn't just about liking the reflection in the mirror or feeling better in your clothes. As metabolic rates begin to shift and slow down, weight gain, especially as we age, puts us at a higher risk of developing an endocrine disorder. Shifting to a diet that focuses on wholesome, plant-based foods provides a remedy.

Another point about plant-based eating for hormonal balance that I think is very important is how eating animal foods can affect the endocrine system. Animal products contain different types of hormones, and choosing grass-fed from your local farmer isn't always a guarantee that your meat, eggs, dairy, etc., won't result in hormonal imbalance. We can refer back to a little earlier when we briefly discussed EDCs. Remember that bit about chemicals being found in water, air, and soil? Farm animals naturally ingest or inhale these toxins, which are delivered to you through your dietary choices.

This problem becomes even worse when we stop to look at where most Americans are sourcing their animal-based foods. The average grocery store sells meat and dairy that has been mass-produced, meaning you can expect more hormones and more chemicals that are known endocrine disruptors.

If we want to look at this most simplistically, adopting a plant-based lifestyle to support hormonal health isn't just about what whole foods do support your health. It's also about moving away from foods that break down your health and disrupt hormonal balance.

A Look at the Best Plant-Based Foods for Hormones

Personally, one of my favorite things is walking into a market that's bursting with fresh, organic produce. I look at all the different colors and my mind immediately begins thinking of ways to enjoy all these foods in their natural glory. I know this isn't the same for everyone.

If you've eaten a mostly SAD diet for your entire life, moving past a few basics in the produce department can be intimidating. Which foods should you eat to support hormonal health?

Which ones are high in the nutrients you may be deficient in? Which ones will your family eat, and what the heck is this weird looking thing anyway?

There's also the very serious issue of a scarcity of fresh, whole foods in some areas. Not everyone has access to a colorful harvest in their local grocery store. Learning about these foods, discovering how to eat them, and learning to love them can be a journey. You might be someone who feels they have a lot to learn but I want you to know that this journey can be incredible and very rewarding.

Now, if you're overwhelmed (and even if you're not) it's always easier to have a starting point. Here I'm providing a list of my favorite plant-based foods for hormonal health. If you don't know where to begin, start here.

Mushrooms

It seems everyone I know has either a love em' or hate em' relationship with mushrooms. If you're not already a fan, I ask you to reconsider. Mushrooms are incredible. They're one of the few natural, non-fortified sources of vitamin D, which is essential for controlling thyroid hormone production – although you're not going to get enough vitamin D from mushrooms alone, so get some sunshine and take a supplement if necessary.

Mushrooms are also being studied for their anti-cancer properties and their ability to potentially slow or kill cancer cells (National Cancer Institute). Not bad for little fungi.

Brazil nuts

Brazil nuts make my list for two reasons. First, they're delicious. Second, they're rich in selenium, a mineral that helps to activate enzymes that stimulate thyroid hormone production. Eat them every day but don't go overboard. While they contain heart-healthy fatty acids, they're also calorically dense.

Anti-Inflammatory Fruits and Vegetables

Except for food sensitivities, it's hard to find anything belonging to the fruit and vegetable family that's not going to support hormonal balance in some way. Starchy vegetables and certain fruits that are high in sugar may be off-limits for people with certain health conditions, like diabetes, but generally speaking, all fruits and vegetables are great options.

Anti-inflammatory fruits and vegetables are even better. These foods prevent inflammation within the body, which is key for keeping hormone production in check. A few of the best anti-inflammatory fruits and vegetables for endocrine health include:

- Berries – blueberries, blackberries, strawberries
- Broccoli
- Avocados
- Green tea
- Turmeric
- Bell peppers
- Cherries

- Tomatoes (unless you have a nightshade sensitivity)

Whole Grains, Nuts, Seeds, and Beans

These plant-based foods provide protein and fiber, both of which are important for your health. For endocrine health, these foods are anti-inflammatory and help regulate hormone overproduction by keeping blood glucose levels balanced.

Foods Rich in Omega-3 and Omega-6 Fatty Acids

You're probably already familiar with these foods as being ones that contain good fats. Olive oil, hemp seeds, flaxseed, walnuts, edamame, and kidney beans are a few examples. Eating foods that are rich in Omega-3 and Omega-6 fatty acids helps to support healthy hypothalamus function.

Foods Containing Vitamins B5 and B6

These two members of the B vitamin family support the pineal gland, helping it produce and release melatonin. If your internal body clock feels like it's ready for a reset, try increasing your consumption of foods like whole grain rice, couscous, potatoes, mushrooms, and sunflower seeds.

Organic Whenever Possible

The chemicals used in traditional farming practices are destructive to endocrine health. I urge you to choose organic produce whenever it's possible. If you have limited access to organic produce or are working with a budget that might not support a fully organic, plant-based diet, start by choosing organic when purchasing fruits and vegetables that make it onto the Environmental Watch Group's dirty dozen list.

CHAPTER SUMMARY

In this chapter, we've talked about the specific disorders that can arise when the endocrine system is out of balance. We've also discussed the main causes of endocrine disorders, including both those we each have control over and the ones we don't. Plant-based foods work therapeutically on multiple levels to bring about healing and hormonal balance. Specifically, we've discussed:

- Common health conditions, including diabetes, hypothyroidism, and PCOS all fall under the umbrella of endocrine disorders
- Symptoms of endocrine disorder include fatigue, weight changes, vision changes, headaches, and depression, just to name a few
- Not all causes of endocrine disorders, such as genetics,

are within our control. Still, dietary adaptations can help us regain healthy endocrine function

- Certain plant-based foods, including the ones mentioned in this chapter, are more effective in creating hormonal balance.

In the next chapter, we're going to talk more about the importance of hormonal harmony. This will include looking closely at each gland of the endocrine system and how to restore balance

3

THE IMPORTANCE OF HORMONAL HARMONY

The endocrine system regulates the hormones that control so many physiological processes. I truly believe that if more people understood the importance of balanced and healthy endocrine function, it might lead to less of the chronic disease and discomfort that we see today.

What I find to be so amazing about the endocrine system is the synergy that's constantly working within it. The endocrine system is responsible for growth and development, reproductive health, responding to injury and chronic stress, regulating metabolism, energy levels, sleep patterns, and keeping the body in a perfect state of homeostasis, or internal equilibrium, the entire time.

There is no way that any singular gland could accomplish this on its own. Synergy and harmony between each gland of the endocrine system are essential for proper functioning. In this chapter, we're going to go much deeper into what each gland of the endocrine system is and the role it plays in your health and wellbeing. One of the key points that I hope you pick up on is how each gland is directly dependent on at least one other. It's a fascinating system and an example of teamwork at its finest.

Another goal I have for you in this chapter is to begin planting the seed that you have the power to take control of your hormonal health. We don't often realize the broad effects that hormone imbalance has on our bodies, and we suffer silently as a result. We think that what we are experiencing is normal, just typical stuff that comes with aging or the stress of working and having a family or simply not having enough time for a little R&R.

In reality, all these symptoms you've been experiencing are very real, and this means that there is a real solution for them. Those chronic headaches that return every evening might be related to stress, but the reason you're continually battling them is that your endocrine system is unbalanced.

The fatigue, malaise, and foggy brain that you chalk up to be overworked are signs of an endocrine disturbance. The irregular, painful periods, the muscle aches, the anxiety, and depression – all of it has roots in an endocrine system that isn't functioning as optimally as it needs to be.

These are the signals your body is sending out to you that something is amiss, that it's time to do something before you're faced with more serious health issues.

I'm such a fan of plant-based nutrition and gentle lifestyle adjustments for hormonal health because these small steps affect your entire endocrine system in such a major way. There's a saying that goes something like "if you can affect or reach just one person, you've made a difference". I like to apply this same concept to endocrine health. If you make a dietary or lifestyle change that initially affects just one gland, you're supporting hormonal harmony and synergy throughout the entire system. It's all connected, and you can make powerful, life-impacting changes to your health.

Major Glands of the Endocrine System

I feel that it's impossible to understand how diet and lifestyle choices can affect your health without a solid foundation of understanding what each gland of the endocrine system does, and its role in your overall health and well-being. In truth, the endocrine system is more complex than we could ever thoroughly cover in a single chapter of a book. After all, some people devote their careers and years of education, to learning how and why the endocrine system functions as it does.

I understand completely that any type of complex medical knowledge can be overwhelming to process, especially if you're just looking for a simple answer and simple solutions. Still, I feel that knowledge is one of the most important tools you can have for improving your health.

My goal here is to present you with a wealth of information about the glands of the endocrine system, and how they influence your overall health. I think this is key to feeling empowered and in control of your health. I also think it is important to understand the hormone-related issues, that you thought were beyond your control without medical or pharmaceutical intervention, can be alleviated with nutritional and lifestyle support.

Here is what I feel is the most important information on the glands of the endocrine system, and how each contributes more broadly to your health.

Hypothalamus – Key Communicator Between the Endocrine and Nervous System

The hypothalamus is small but mighty. This small gland, located near the central area of the brain, has the important job of serving as the link between the entire endocrine system and the nervous system. The hypothalamus produces hormones that are crucial players in many nervous system processes.

The hypothalamus is like the control center that keeps your body in a state of homeostasis – in other words, everything is balanced just as it should be. The hypothalamus is solely responsible for stimulating many essential body processes through the release of hormones.

The hypothalamus is important in the regulation of body temperature, electrolyte balance, sleep regulation, heart rate, blood pressure, metabolism, appetite, and weight maintenance – and this is all just the tip of the iceberg.

The Hypothalamus and Its Hormones

So, the question is, what happens when the hypothalamus is out of balance? It's one tiny, little gland. Can it really cause that much damage if it becomes out of balance? To answer those questions, it's important to first understand that the hypothalamus is involved in the production and regulation of a great number of hormones, each playing a significant role in your overall health in some way.

The role of the hypothalamus in hormone regulation is largely connected to its relationship with the pituitary gland. The hypothalamus and pituitary gland work hand in hand.

The nervous system sends out signals, which are received by the hypothalamus. The hypothalamus then serves as the messenger, telling the pituitary glands to either amp up or slow down the secretion of hormones.

A single hiccup in the communication train and any number of the hormones released by the pituitary gland can become unbalanced. The hypothalamus and the pituitary gland have their own delicate "ecosystem" that needs to be balanced to function properly. You can't talk about the health of the hypothalamus without also talking about pituitary health, and vice versa.

The involvement of the hypothalamus in hormonal health is expansive. Here is just a quick rundown of the main hormones that are produced, secreted, and regulated by hypothalamus involvement.

Oxytocin: We'll start with oxytocin because it's one that many people have at least heard of. It's often referred to as the "love hormone", and with valid reason. When we have close, embracing contact with another person – think a hug, cuddle, or skin to skin contact with a newborn, the body automatically releases more oxytocin into the system.

Oxytocin is thought to factor so heavily into our emotional responses, that psychologists are beginning to look more seriously at how this hormone creates feelings of trust and belonging. This, however, isn't the extent of oxytocin's role (DeAngelis).

Oxytocin, which is produced by the hypothalamus and released by the pituitary gland, is a crucial hormone for women's reproductive health. It stimulates uterine contractions before, during, and after childbirth, and signals the "letdown" of breast milk in response to a suckling infant. Oxytocin is essential for mother-infant bonding.

If the hypothalamus is unbalanced and not producing oxytocin as it should, your body can suffer a range of consequences. Oxytocin is involved in body temperature control and sleep cycle regulation. If either of these processes strays off course, it can produce a spider-web effect of symptoms.

Growth hormone-releasing hormone: This hormone, more often referred to as GHRH, is vital for the proper growth and development of children. Its release stimulates growth hormones in the pituitary gland. For children who experience precocious puberty, this hormone plays a role in the associated rapid growth spurts and sometimes shorter stature.

The importance of GHRH doesn't stop after puberty. It's essential to bone growth and bone structure, maintaining or building muscle mass, body fat distribution, and affects protein, fat, and carbohydrate metabolism.

Gonadotrophin-releasing hormone: This hormone has one very important role. It's produced by the hypothalamus, and then sends signals to the pituitary gland to secrete other hormones that keep the reproductive glands (ovaries and testes) functioning properly. You're likely to see gonadotropin-releasing hormone referenced as GnRH (so much easier to say!), and without it, reproduction isn't possible.

Antidiuretic hormone: This little-known hormone is essential for proper kidney function. It supports the absorption of water into the blood by the kidneys. If you have too little ADH in your system, troublesome symptoms like frequent urination, dehydration, and excessive thirst can present themselves. An excessive amount of this hormone is sometimes associated with more serious health conditions, including cancers of the bladder, pancreas, and lung. It may also be present in higher amounts in people with epilepsy and other serious health conditions.

ADH is also important for metabolic regulation and for building a healthy immune system. It partners with the pituitary gland in a chain response that eventually leads to the release of corticosteroids by the adrenals.

Prolactin related hormones: Referred to as either prolactin inhibiting hormone (PIH) or prolactin-releasing hormone (PRH) is involved in the lactation process for nursing mothers. The release of PRH signals to the pituitary gland that it's time to produce prolactin, which stimulates breast milk production. On the opposite end of the spectrum, the release of PIH inhibits milk production.

Thyrotropin-releasing hormone: TRH is a hormone that stimulates and activates the thyroid, which is key for balancing all the thyroid hormones that regulate essential body processes like metabolism, growth, and development.

Signs and Symptoms of Hypothalamus Imbalance

Like any of the other glands in the endocrine system, an imbalance of the hypothalamus can be caused by a variety of factors. For some, genetic influences are the cause behind hypothalamus dysfunction. For others, the causes can be quite varied – ranging from malnutrition and eating disorders to infection.

This is one of those scenarios where the underlying cause of hypothalamus dysfunction can't be assessed until the symptoms become quite noticeable. Here are a few of the ways that imbalances in the hypothalamus, and the hormones it produces, can manifest itself.

- Sleep disturbance
- Extreme fatigue
- Mood swings
- Anxiety and depression
- Irritability
- Fluctuations in libido
- Digestive disturbances
- Frequent thirst
- Sensitivity to heat
- Itchiness that can't be attributed to other factors

Healing the Hypothalamus

Depending on the source of hypothalamus involvement, it is entirely possible to restore balance through a shift in nutritional habits. Shunning foods that are high in saturated fats and processed sugars and replacing them with foods that are nourishing and healing, especially those that contain omega-3 fatty acids, is a good start. The hypothalamus responds positively to foods like walnuts, flaxseed, green leafy vegetables, and foods rich in both B vitamins and vitamin C.

Pituitary – The Master Gland

The pituitary gland is a perfect example of small but mighty. The pituitary gland is a tiny, pea-sized structure that sits at the base of the brain. Its location isn't far from the hypothalamus, which isn't surprising considering how these two glands work so closely together.

Just like the hypothalamus sends signals to the pituitary gland, the pituitary controls many of the functions carried out by other glands of the endocrine system.

Because the pituitary functions somewhat as command central in the endocrine system, it's often referred to as the master gland. Think of the pituitary as the main on-sight manager of the endocrine system that keeps everything running smoothly, and the hypothalamus as the regional manager that offers guidance and insight based on the pituitary's reporting.

Pituitary function is directly connected to what we call target glands and organs. These include the adrenals, thyroid, ovaries, testes, and kidneys. Breasts and female reproductive organs are also dependent on pituitary involvement.

What I find interesting about the pituitary gland is that the hormones produced by it do not continually flow through the body. Instead, they're released cyclically, about once every one-to-three hours. I enjoy this factoid about this little gland because it reinforces the need for regular cycles in our lives. Sleep, wake, work, play – all in proper amounts and a routine our bodies can rely on. The pituitary glands show us that no matter how powerful we are, rest is essential for optimal performance.

I've mentioned sleep and its importance for overall health and wellbeing. Your body naturally has a circadian rhythm that works as an internal timer, determining when you wake, when you sleep, and when hormones are released. Some of these hormones are released by the pituitary gland. For example, the levels of the hormone prolactin are higher during the night while you're sleeping, peaking before you wake, and then tapering off throughout the day. When your sleep patterns are off, it disrupts your circadian rhythm, having a direct impact on hormonal health.

The pituitary gland also works hard to regulate hormone production and release in ways besides a daily fluctuation. Women, from puberty through menopause, rely on the pituitary gland to release hormones on a regular cycle for reproductive health. If the pituitary gland isn't releasing reproductive hormones on schedule, she is likely to experience problems with infertility. Men, and their reproductive health, are also affected by pituitary deficiencies that interfere with the production of sex hormones.

As we age, the pituitary gland remains important. Cardiovascular disease and osteoporosis are two age-related health concerns with potential pituitary involvement. Osteoporosis or low bone mass affects approximately 44 million people in the United States, representing about 55% of adults over the age of

50 (International Osteoporosis Foundation). An imbalance in the performance of the pituitary gland can result in hormonal deficiencies, which are suspected to be contributing factors in the development of osteoporosis (Bolanowski, Halupczok, & Jawiarczyk-Przybyłowska). Protecting your bones isn't as much about drinking a glass of cow milk each day, as it is supporting healthy pituitary function through a diet packed with plant-based nutrients.

Because the hypothalamus and pituitary glands were so close together, many of the hormones affected by the pituitary gland are the same ones listed under the hypothalamus. For example, the hormones that are produced or stored in the anterior (front) lobe of the pituitary gland include prolactin and growth hormone, as well as the thyroid-stimulating hormone, luteinizing hormone, follicle-stimulating hormone (important for reproduction), and adrenocorticotropin, which stimulates cortisol production. The posterior, or back portion of the pituitary gland controls oxytocin and antidiuretic hormones.

Are you feeling like a medical student yet? The endocrine system is so complex, this is only the beginning but a solid foundation in understanding how it works is essential for hormonal health and balance.

Signs and Symptoms of Pituitary Imbalance

Unfortunately, we're often quick to dismiss many of the key indicators of endocrine imbalance as common everyday maladies. We associate them with stress, lack of self-care, or simply growing older. This is true for many of the signs and symptoms of pituitary dysfunction. Here are a few of the main symptoms to be aware of.

- Sleep disturbances
- Headaches
- Fatigue
- General weakness
- Infertility
- Irregular periods
- Erectile dysfunction
- Mood swings
- Depression
- Weight gain not associated with dietary or lifestyle changes
- Memory decline
- Elevated blood pressure
- Lactation not associated with pregnancy or breastfeeding
- Excessive hair growth

Healing the Pituitary Gland

Adopting and maintaining a balanced diet is so important for pituitary health. This is especially true for children, whose growth can be negatively impacted by malnutrition. When I speak of malnutrition here, I'm not just referring to a lack of food, such as what we see in less affluent nations, and the most underprivileged areas of the United States. I'm also referring to a diet of refined, processed foods that lack real nutritional value – something that has become all too common for our youth.

Eating a diet that is filled with fresh fruits, vegetables, and whole grains is thought to be effective for protecting the pituitary gland from disease. You want to look for the most nutrient-dense foods that are also high in fiber. Omega-3s are also important for pituitary health, as is cutting back on fatty meats, refined sugars, and sodium.

Thyroid – Miraculous Butterfly

The thyroid is a butterfly-shaped gland that is found in the neck, rather low in the front. While the thyroid gland sits in the front, along the windpipe, it isn't something you can normally feel when you run a hand along your neck. When something is going on with the thyroid gland that causes it to swell, it does become noticeable through touch and often a visible bump on the neck.

The thyroid gland is one of those that most people learn about in basic biology and anatomy classes in high school or college but that is about the extent of familiarity most of us have – that is until it gives us a reason to stand up and take notice. The thyroid doesn't produce the number of hormones that the hypothalamus and pituitary glands do, but its involvement in the body is still crucial and far-reaching.

The thyroid directly influences major organs, including the heart, brain, kidneys, and liver. The thyroid also plays a role in the health of your skin, which is your largest and most often underappreciated organ. Without a properly functioning thyroid, you're going to have problems.

Your thyroid is responsible for regulating metabolism, but not just in the way you're thinking. The thyroid regulates cell metabolism, which is to say it controls how fast or slow your cells work. Your thyroid creates, stores, and releases two hormones called T3 and T4. Of these, T4 is more abundantly produced by the thyroid. T4, once it leaves the thyroid and reaches the cells of other tissues and organs, converts to T3 where it is most needed. Your thyroid is an incredibly, fine-tuned machine.

When the thyroid overproduces hormones, it revs up cellular metabolism, causing them to work faster than normal. We call this hyperthyroidism. On the other end of thyroid dysfunction is when too little thyroid hormones are released, causing cellular metabolism to become sluggish. We refer to this condition as hypothyroidism.

At first, it can be difficult to fully grasp the effects of fast or slow cellular metabolism. I mean, as long as things are actually working in the cells, what does it matter if it progresses a little faster or slower than normal? Trust me when I say that cellular metabolism makes a tremendous difference.

As an example, let's look at an infant who has been born with thyroid dysfunction that slows cellular metabolism. Now consider that the brain is among the thyroid's target organs. A slow functioning thyroid is going to inhibit the cellular processes needed for proper neurodevelopment, which is something that is already so incredibly fragile during the earliest months and years of life.

For those of us that have made it a bit further (ok, a lot further) in life, an overactive thyroid that speeds up cellular metabolism in the heart can lead to cardiac issues, including palpitations and stress from a rapid heart rate. Can thyroid disturbances affect your ability to lose or maintain weight? You bet but the effects that you can't see or immediately feel can be far more detrimental to your long-term health.

One more important thing to note about the thyroid is its involvement in autoimmune disorders. An autoimmune disorder is a condition where the body recognizes its own tissues as invasive pathogens and attacks them with an overactive immune response. Two common types of autoimmune diseases affect the thyroid – Hashimoto Disease and Graves Disease.

While there are certainly many factors that contribute to autoimmune disease, and so much is still unknown, diet can have a very strong and direct impact on the severity and life impact that these diseases have on your health.

Signs and Symptoms of Thyroid Disease and Dysfunction

Because the thyroid can become both overactive and underactive, pinpointing symptoms of imbalance is difficult until the disease reaches the point that has a more significant impact on one's health.

Signs of an overactive thyroid include:

- Hair loss
- Menstrual irregularities, especially light or absent menstrual periods.
- Shakiness or trembling
- Irritability and mood disturbances
- Anxiety
- Profuse sweating
- Sensitivity to heat

Signs of an underactive thyroid include:

- Sleep disturbances
- Excessive fatigue
- Dry skin
- Mood disturbances and depression
- Issues with memory, focus, and concentration
- Menstrual irregularities, especially heavy periods and periods that come more frequently than normal

- Muscle and joint discomfort
- Chills
- Sensitivity to cold

Healing the Thyroid Gland

What's unique about the thyroid gland is that it is dependent upon one crucial mineral to function properly – iodine. Natural food sources of iodine include fish and seafood, dairy products, and certain grain products. This presents a bit of a challenge for plant-based eaters, but there are ways to get adequate iodine in your diet, even if you choose to forgo seafood and dairy.

Iodized salt is a primary source of iodine, no matter which type of diet you're following. If you're low on natural sources of iodine in your diet, make sure to choose a table salt that has been iodized. Sea salt and other types of coarse salts usually haven't been iodized. There's also a delicate balance that needs to be kept here. Most people are not hurting due to lack of iodized salt in their diets and overdoing it on sodium can lead to bigger problems.

If you're on a salt-restricted diet, whether it's for personal or medical reasons, you can skip the salt and get your iodine in supplement form. Many complete vitamin supplements contain iodine, so make sure to take a look at the label of any nutritional supplement you may be taking to ensure you don't over-consume iodine by taking unnecessary supplements.

Due to the thyroid's involvement in auto-immune diseases, following some type of auto-immune protocol with your diet can help prevent, minimize, or in some cases heal thyroid-related auto-immune disease. Every auto-immune protocol that I've seen has included a focus on anti-inflammatory foods. A plant-based diet that eliminates unhealthy fats, sugars, processed ingredients, and dietary toxins is one of the most effective ways to control an inflammatory response.

Adrenals – Fight or Flight, and So Much More

I find it fascinating that the glands of the endocrine system are so small yet have such a broad impact on health. The Adrenal glands are no exception. You have two small adrenal glands, each one located on top of a kidney. Your adrenals each have two lobes, and together they are responsible for influencing several hormonally controlled functions and help control your body's stress response, metabolism, immune health, and sexual function.

The two different lobes of the adrenal gland are called the adrenal cortex and adrenal medulla. One of the most important hormones secreted by the adrenal cortex is cortisol. Cortisol has a bit of a bad reputation, at no fault of its own. When your body perceives a threat, it has a natural response system, which includes the production of cortisol to help it adapt to the perceived threat.

Stress can come in a range of forms, from legitimately fearing for your safety, to being overworked, emotionally drained, and constantly feeling at least a low level (if not more) of daily stress. Cortisol stimulates the body's fight or flight response, which is absolutely essential in dealing with stress. In a perfect world, your body would create cortisol to help you deal with stress, then levels would decline, and all would be good.

Considering our modern lifestyle, this usually isn't what happens.

When balanced, cortisol is important for regulating blood pressure, metabolism, quenching inflammation, regulating blood sugar, and promoting healthy sleep cycles. It helps your body by providing a surge of energy when dealing with stress but also helping you rest and recover after the event. The problem is that many of us are experiencing stress at such a constant pace that cortisol levels never back down.

Instead, it keeps getting pumped through our bodies at levels that are higher than normal, even when no immediate threat is present. This stresses the adrenal glands and causes a range of health issues, including weight gain, heart disease, sleep disturbances, mood disorders, and difficulty concentrating on anything for any period of time. High levels of cortisol are also associated with the accumulation of adipose tissue around the midsection (one of the most dangerous places to gain weight), which explains why you might notice your clothes fitting a little tighter when you're under stress.

So, cortisol is a major hormone that's regulated by the adrenals but it's not the only one. The adrenal cortex is also responsible for aldosterone, which helps regulate the pH of your blood, and a small amount of female and male sex hormones. The adrenal medulla is responsible for the production of epinephrine and norepinephrine, which are also key players in the fight or flight response. When the adrenals aren't working efficiently, they can't respond properly to stress.

There are specific health issues that directly affect the adrenal glands. These include Addison's Disease (adrenal insufficiency), Cushing's Syndrome, benign tumors, adrenal cancer, and congenital adrenal hyperplasia. There's one more condition affecting the adrenals called adrenal fatigue, a condition that the medical community doesn't entirely back.

Understanding Adrenal Fatigue

Adrenal fatigue, which is not recognized by the medical community as a valid diagnosis, is a term used to describe a set of non-specific health-related symptoms. It's much like chronic fatigue syndrome in the way that those who suffer from it experience very real symptoms that seem unrelated to each other yet getting help from the medical community often feels fruitless.

People who experience adrenal fatigue can have symptoms that include general malaise and fatigue, sleep disturbances, widespread body aches and pains, digestive issues, headaches, anxiety, and nervousness. If you were to go to the standard doctor with this list of symptoms, they'd probably do a few blood tests to rule out more serious health conditions, and then send you on your way with advice on how to reduce stress and get better sleep. Adrenal function may never even enter the picture.

If a doctor does recognize your symptoms as possibly being adrenal related, a blood test that measures adrenal function still might not give much a clue as to what's going on. With adrenal fatigue, it's suggested that the adrenal glands are under a level of constant stress, which affects their ability to perform but not to the extent that it would appear obvious on normal test markers.

Signs and Symptoms of Adrenal Disease

When adrenal dysfunction progresses beyond the point of adrenal fatigue, a person might experience a vast range of symptoms, including:

- Extreme fatigue
- Low blood pressure
- Low blood sugar levels
- Dizziness
- Excessive perspiration
- Digestive upset, including nausea and vomiting
- Weight fluctuations
- Widespread muscle and joint pain
- Unexplained skin discoloration and darkening
- Menstrual irregularities
- Cravings for salty foods

Healing the Adrenal Glands Through Nutrition

The key to supporting adrenal health through diet and nutrition is eliminating foods that place additional stress on your endocrine system. Think along the line of whole foods, with minimal processing and added ingredients to spark inflammation or interfere with your body's natural healing processes.

Eating a balanced diet of natural, whole foods, regular exercise, and stress relief are key to supporting adrenal health. Any lifestyle change you make that reduces stress, and its impact on your body, is a winning point for adrenal health.

Pineal Gland – Your Body's Internal Time Clock

The pineal gland, which is this tiny pea-shaped gland that is nestled in the brain, is still a bit of an enigma. When it comes to medical research and study of the endocrine system, the pineal gland has come in last, being the final gland to be discovered and studied. This means that there is still much we don't know about the pineal gland, how it functions, and its overall supporting role in endocrine health.

What we do know about the pineal gland is that it's responsible for regulating at least one very important hormone – melatonin.

Melatonin is a name that many people recognize from the vitamin and supplement aisle. Pop melatonin in the evening to have sweet dreams and restful sleep. Melatonin as a supplement has become popular because our sleep-wake cycles are so disrupted. For the many people who work second or third shifts, it's next to impossible to follow your body's natural sleep/wake patterns, so your body adjusts, often putting additional stress on the pineal gland.

It isn't just working odd hours that's to blame. So many people choose to trade sleep in favor of a few minutes of quiet time at the end of the day. Time with no responsibilities, to do whatever they want, sans kids or obligations. For many night owls, staying up into the wee hours of the morning is a sanity saver.

It might seem like a decent trade-off, but your natural body clock is sure to be in disagreement. When we purposefully shift our sleep patterns, we disrupt our natural circadian rhythm, which can be extremely difficult to return to normal. One of the main symptoms of pineal disruption is difficulty regulating sleep-wake cycles, including chronic insomnia and the associated health-related side effects that come with it.

While melatonin's function in regulating the body's circadian rhythm is well-known, melatonin also plays an important role in female reproductive health. Research on melatonin suggests that it blocks the secretion of gonadotropins. Gonadotropins include the follicle-stimulating hormone (FSH) and luteinizing hormone (LH) that assist in both the development and functioning of reproductive glands. In females, FSH and LH are factors in ovulation and ovarian quality concerning fertility.

When these levels aren't what they should be, infertility and menstrual irregularities are common side effects

Melatonin is also thought to offer a degree of protection against certain types of cardiovascular diseases, such as hypertension and atherosclerosis. One tiny pea-shaped gland, and one primary hormone, but such an incredible effect on one's health.

Restoring Balance in the Pineal Gland

Restoring balance in the pineal gland almost always involves some type of lifestyle adjustments that promote the regulation of melatonin. This might include looking for ways to eliminate the need to stay up late, remove distractions that keep you awake at night, taking a look at any medication to determine if they could be disruptive to your sleep/wake cycle, avoiding foods that cause digestive upset, and addressing any causes of stress that might be contributing to wakefulness.

The pineal gland is also prone to calcification, which can interfere with proper function. Including certain plant-based foods in your diet can help detoxify and prevent, reduce, or eliminate pineal calcification. A few foods that are suggested for detoxifying the pineal gland include apple cider vinegar, beets, green leafy vegetables, and small amounts of iodized salt, or foods that have been fortified with iodine.

Ovaries and Testes – Reproductive Command Central

The ovaries and testes are the reproductive glands of the endocrine system. They produce the sex hormones that are responsible for puberty, sexual maturity, reproduction, and eventually menopause in women. In the simplest terms, the human race would cease to exist if it weren't for the ovaries and testes. They really are that important.

Moving away from the universal importance of the reproductive glands, we can shift our focus to how they affect a person's health individually.

In males, the testes are the primary source of sex hormones. The testes are located in the scrotum, and release sex hormones called androgens – one of the most well-known being testosterone. We often associate testosterone with uber-masculinity but its role is much more complex.

Both males and females produce some level of testosterone, with males producing more. One of testosterone's primary roles involves sexual/reproductive health but the hormone is also essential for metabolic regulation, insulin sensitivity, body composition, and some research suggests that it's also related to heart health and bone density in females.

In males, the symptoms of testosterone imbalance can include delayed onset of puberty, sexual dysfunction, loss of libido, overactive libido, obesity, loss of muscle mass, fatigue, and hair loss. While testosterone is produced by other parts of the endocrine system in females, symptoms of imbalance can include menstrual irregularities, infertility, acne, excessive hair growth or hair loss, weight gain, and mood disturbances.

During puberty in males, the testes signal the onset of puberty. When the testes are functioning properly, they determine when puberty occurs, and how it affects the male's body – including growth, vocal changes, and the growth of facial hair. At a certain point in puberty, the testes, and the pineal gland function together to determine when the male begins to make sperm for reproduction.

In females, ovaries are the reproductive glands of the endocrine system. They are primarily responsible for regulating two hormones called estrogen and progesterone. Each is important during puberty and for the regulation of a female's menstrual cycle. Once a female moves beyond puberty, these hormones play critical roles in fertility, pregnancy, and menopause.

In females, we are continually learning more about how estrogen and progesterone work in the body and the effects of these two hormones becoming unbalanced. For example, estrogen dominance is a hormone-related issue that is becoming more common. Normally, there is a balance between estrogen and progesterone, barring pregnancy, at least until a woman begins to near menopause.

Estrogen dominance isn't necessarily the excessive production of estrogen, although that can be involved. Instead, it refers more to a decline in progesterone levels which disrupts the synergistic balance between the two hormones. Estrogen dominance can create unpleasant symptoms such as insomnia, weight gain, mood disturbances, and low sex drive but it can also create a situation where a woman is more at risk of health conditions that are influenced by estrogen levels, such as heart disease and certain cancers.

The ovaries are complex members of the endocrine system. They work with other glands in the release of reproductive hormones that stimulate the maturation and release of egg cells during ovulation, and they accomplish this repeatedly, with a fairly predictable monthly cycle.

The degree to which the testes and ovaries function is something that fluctuates throughout our lifetimes. Men experience a natural decline in testosterone as they age, and a woman's hormones begin to fluctuate widely as she nears menopause, creating some very uncomfortable, and sometimes life-altering, symptoms.

Is Hormone Replacement the Answer?

While some men choose testosterone supplements or steroids to enhance their testosterone levels as they age, hormonal replacement isn't nearly as common with men as it is with women. Hormonal therapy is frequently prescribed by the medical community to help ease the discomforts of menstruation and menopause.

Whether or not a person chooses hormonal therapy is of course a personal one, but it's also a decision that should be made with great care and knowledge. There is an ever-growing amount of research indicating that hormone replacement therapy can create significant, serious health concerns with long term use. We're talking about major health issues here, like heart disease and an elevated risk of hormone-dependent cancers.

There is a definite risk/benefit profile that should be weighed and considered before jumping on board with hormone therapy. What I've found when working with clients that are dealing with wild hormonal fluctuations that so desperately want relief but understandably want to avoid hormone treatments, is that simple changes to diet and lifestyle can often bring about the relief that they're looking for.

Diet can either work for or against you in terms of hormonal health, especially regarding hormones regulated by the ovaries and testes. Many animal-based foods, including meats and dairy, contain added hormones that interfere with how your hormones are produced and synthesized. Foods that are calorically dense but nutritionally void lead to weight gain, which directly affects reproductive hormone balance.

Processed foods, toxic ingredients, and a diet void of any real amount of fiber are like a death sentence for optimal hormonal health. One could easily argue that age-related hormonal fluctuations are normal and tolerable. What isn't normal is the way our hormones react at these transitional times in our lives due to dietary and lifestyle factors that negatively affect hormonal balance for potentially years to come.

CHAPTER SUMMARY

In this chapter, we've looked at the importance of hormonal harmony – both overall and within each gland of the endocrine system. We had a chance to look at each gland specifically, discussing what happens when it becomes out of balance, along with what can be done to return each member of the endocrine system to a balanced state. Specifically, we've discussed:

- Each gland of the endocrine systems plays a critical role in your health
- Endocrine imbalances will manifest themselves differently depending on which gland is affected
- An individualized approach is needed to restore hormonal balance, including dietary adaptations
- Hormone replacement is an option for some but it's a choice that should be made with a great deal of thought and knowledge.

In the next chapter, we're going to focus on how plant-based nutrition works to treat the root cause of imbalance, rather than just the symptoms. In discussing this, we're going to look more closely at autoimmune diseases that arise as a manifestation of hormonal imbalance.

TREATING THE SOURCE, NOT THE SYMPTOMS

I find it interesting that a primary focus of traditional medicine is to treat the symptoms, sometimes without giving much thought to the underlying conditions. After all, if you treat the source of the problem, won't the symptoms cease to exist?

This may be true but we're the instant gratification culture. How many times have you reached for an over the counter pain reliever to soothe a throbbing headache without considering that the cause of the headache might be eyestrain, stress, lack of sleep, or allergies? It's okay to want quick relief from anything uncomfortable or disruptive to our lives but we should be equally focused on healing what ails us.

Think of it this way. If your smoke detector were to go off, would you just turn it off or rip the batteries out without first looking to see if you could find a cause for the alarm? If you did find the cause, wouldn't you at least attempt to put out the fire or call your local emergency team in to do it for you, rather than just quiet the alarm while ignoring the real problem?

Of course, you would but this is not what we're doing when we look only at treating the symptoms and not the source. You might have quieted the symptoms for now but inside you've got a fire raging out of control that needs to be addressed before it burns through your entire body.

With my clients, I've repeatedly seen evidence that we're a society that thinks if the symptoms are better, then so is the underlying cause. Taking ibuprofen might take the back pain away for a bit but it doesn't heal the strained muscle that's causing it. In some cases, the source may heal on its own but there are many times when the source problem is chronic and systemic and isn't going anywhere unless it is addressed specifically.

Such is the case with autoimmune disease, which is why I've decided to take a chapter of this book and focus on autoimmune conditions and what causes them. I also chose to go a little further in-depth into autoimmune diseases because the root cause of them is relatively unknown. We don't fully understand what triggers an autoimmune disorder, but we do know that inflammation is present in all of them, and that a continual, chronic inflammatory response is what leads to a long list of autoimmune disorder side effects that the medical community is so eager to fix.

I'd like to suggest that in addition to easing the symptoms of autoimmune disease that we work diligently to treat the source of the problem, which in this case is inflammation. As we talk more about autoimmune disorders and their common thread of inflammation, I want you to keep in mind the effects that inflammation has on the endocrine system and hormone production.

Several autoimmune disorders affect the endocrine system directly but for the most part, I want to look at autoimmune disorders with a broader lens and explore the possibilities of reducing inflammation through dietary changes, including adopting a plant-based style of eating.

What Is an Autoimmune Disorder?

Autoimmune disorders are complex and often misunderstood. Currently, we know of at least eighty different autoimmune disorders. Some, like rheumatoid arthritis, are more common and affect more than a million people in the United States alone. Others are rare, affecting a mere handful of individuals worldwide.

We're continually learning more about autoimmune disorders, how they affect the body, and what we can do both medically and holistically to relieve them. In the most basic terms, an autoimmune disorder involves the body's immune system becoming overactive and attacking the body itself, rather than just the unpleasant things that attempt to invade it.

Your immune system is incredibly important, in fact, you wouldn't be alive without it. A healthy immune system stands constant guard against invasions from bacteria, viruses, and all sorts of germs you encounter every single day. As soon as the body senses that any of these invaders are present, it sends out special fighter cells to knock them out.

One would think that having an overactive immune system wouldn't be such a bad thing, but in the case of autoimmune disorders, it is. When a person has an autoimmune disorder, their immune system mistakenly targets parts of itself and releases these things called autoantibodies. You've probably heard of antibodies before but put an "auto" in front of the word, and you have problems.

Antibodies are proteins, and they're among the body's chief lines of defense against pathogens. I'll spare you the long biology lecture here, but your body also has these things called memory cells, which produce antibodies of their own in response to viruses, bacteria, etc. These types of antibodies remember certain pathogens and can recall instantly how to fight them off. This is why you might have a period of immunity to disease after you've been sick.

Autoantibodies are also proteins that act in the same way but in this case, they attack the tissues, organs, and joints of the body, create inflammation, and sometimes damage the area that they attack. There are different types of autoantibodies, with some of them presenting as markers that predict disease before the symptoms of it become obvious.

In some autoimmune disorders, the body singles out and targets just one part of the body. An example of this might be type I diabetes in which the immune system targets the pancreas, although the residual damage extends much further than that. In other types of autoimmune disease, multiple parts of the body are targeted and attacked. These types of disorders are labeled as systemic and end up destroying cells throughout the body. Autoimmune disorders may result in permanent changes, including organ or tissue damage, abnormal growth to tissues or organs, and eventually structural changes that can affect how an organ functions.

As mentioned earlier, there are at least 80 different types of autoimmune diseases that we're currently aware of, and it's estimated that as many as 23.5 million people suffer from autoimmune disorders, just in the United States alone. A list of the most common autoimmune disorders that people are suffering from today would include:

- Addison Disease
- Celiac Disease
- Graves Disease
- Multiple Sclerosis

- Hashimoto Thyroiditis
- Endometriosis
- Crohn's Disease
- Ulcerative Colitis
- Rheumatoid Arthritis
- Type I Diabetes
- Systemic Lupus
- Sjogren Syndrome
- Juvenile Arthritis
- Psoriasis
- Kawasaki Disease
- Vasculitis

The tricky thing about autoimmune disorders is that their cause is largely still a mystery. We don't yet fully understand at this point what it is that causes these misfires in the immune system. While there are no hard and fast rules about who gets an autoimmune disease and who doesn't, it does seem that certain people have a somewhat elevated risk.

For example, women develop autoimmune disorders at a notably higher rate than men. One study looks at the prevalence of autoimmune disease based on gender and found that more than twice as many women than men were affected (Hayter & Cook, 2012). With this, there seems to be a relationship with the onset of autoimmune disease and a woman's childbearing years. Whether this is correlation or causation is yet to be determined but it does pose an interesting question in the role of hormones in autoimmune disease, especially in women.

Other factors seem to influence the occurrence of autoimmune conditions. For instance, lupus is not nearly as common in Caucasians as it is in African Americans, Asian- Americans, and Hispanics. Genetics also seems to play a role in some autoimmune diseases but rather than "passing down" a specific disease through genetic markers, like cystic fibrosis, for example, there seems to be a genetic susceptibility to a range of autoimmune disorders within a genetic line.

Some also suspect that certain autoimmune disorders may be the result of environmental factors. The possibility of bacterial or viral infections playing a role has been explored, as well as exposure to chemicals and toxins. While we don't know what causes autoimmune disorders in everyone that suffers from them, this information does tell us that not everyone is at equal risk and that there may be things we can do on an individual level to further reduce those risks or minimize the severity of an existing autoimmune disorder – including taking steps to build a strong foundation of health through nutritional healing and balanced hormones.

The Relationship Between Diet and Autoimmune Disorder

Each autoimmune disorder uniquely affects the body but we're seeing that the one thing they all have in common is inflammation. There is an increasing body of evidence that an enhanced inflammatory response is associated with autoimmune disorders, as well as chronic disease across the board (Duan, Rao, & Sigdel. 2019). Considering the role of inflammation in chronic disease, it becomes important to look at what we can do to reduce inflammation through lifestyle choices.

There are actually many little things you can do that may have a positive effect on reducing your body's overactive inflammatory response. Exercising and stress reduction are two examples of seemingly small steps that can have a significant influence on inflammation. Both of these things affect hormones that play a role in inflammation. Something you can do that is even more impactful is making shifts in your diet that reduce or eliminate foods that are known to increase inflammatory markers.

Here is where I'm going to say something that might not sit well with some of you hard-core omnivores out there. We know that processed foods, fats, sugars, refined grains, etc. are inflammatory foods. What we're learning is that certain animal-based foods are equal culprits in fueling the type of inflammation that leads to chronic disease, including autoimmune disorders.

One type of food that appears to be an obvious culprit for many is dairy. According to the Arthritis Foundation, there is a potential link between dairy and inflammation, which can make arthritis worse for some people (Paturel). Dairy has also been implicated in abnormal immune responses in susceptible individuals, and it is believed that this may serve as a trigger to certain autoimmune disorders, especially those with neurological involvement.

What makes dairy's involvement in autoimmune disorders more confusing is the fact that some people are highly sensitive to dairy products, while others appear to have no known adverse effects. Notice that I referred to no "known" adverse effects here. It's estimated that as much as 65% of the population has a reduced capacity to digest lactose (NIH). In people of Asian descent, this number is even higher. These numbers represent a number well above the majority threshold and considering that inflammation is common in lactose/dairy sensitivity, it's no surprise that we're suffering more frequently from inflammation-related chronic diseases.

The next thing I want to talk about is animal protein, particularly red meat, and inflammation. The research linking red meat consumption to the onset of autoimmune disorders isn't significant enough to really mention here but there has been ample research into whether consuming animal proteins lead to inflammation and how diet can affect later-onset chronic inflammatory diseases (Rasmussen, Rubin, Stougaard, Tjøn-neland, Stenager, Lund Hetlan, . . . Andersen, 2019).

At this point, a majority of people are familiar with low-carb or keto diets that strongly promote animal proteins as the main source of caloric energy and fats. These diets also restrict carbohydrate intake, even when those carbs come from nutritionally dense sources. The idea being that your body will better utilize stored fat for fuel. There are hordes of people out there who will swear by the results of their keto-style diets, and maybe you're one of them.

I'm not going to argue that eating low carb will help you lose weight because it can. I'm also not going to argue that people with chronic inflammation might feel temporary relief when they embark on this style of diet. Losing weight and staying away from many of the sugary and processed foods that are eliminated with these eating plans are both positives for reducing inflammation. The issue here is that these diets simply aren't meant to support the body nutritionally long term, and we're also learning more about the negative long-term effects these diets can have on one's health.

I want to make the argument here that one of the reasons low-carb and carnivore-centered diets aren't the best for you is because of how the main component of the diet, animal protein, is known to spark systemic inflammation.

For years now, we've been telling people to cut out foods, especially grains that contain gluten, because of the potential for inflammation. If you're someone who truly suffers from a food sensitivity, then you must follow this advice. However, there are many out there that follow this type of advice without fully understanding inflammation and how food plays a role. As a result, we're eliminating foods that are actually anti-inflammatory and replacing them with foods that are known to increase inflammation.

Today, we know that the consumption of red meat is associated with an increase in inflammatory markers, and it honestly doesn't matter if your meat is grass-fed or humanely raised. There are components of the meat itself that work against your body, fuel inflammation, and make conditions like autoimmune disease even worse.

Instead of just shaking my finger and telling you that red and processed meats are bad from an inflammation standpoint, I want to take a minute and explain exactly why this is the case.

The first is something called TMAO (or trimethylamine oxide if we're being technical about it). TMAO is formed after you consume choline, which is found in animal-based protein sources, like muscle tissue. It is 100% completely unnecessary to take in TMAO from dietary sources because your own body is capable of producing what it needs – in the proper amounts. When consumed from dietary sources, TMAO is associated with an increased risk of cardiovascular disease, which just happens to be (you guessed it) an inflammatory health condition.

Next up, are these reactive molecules called AGES, which if you ask me is appropriately named because the inflammation they cause can prematurely age you in so many ways. Seriously though, AGES stands for advanced glycation end products, and they are formed when fats and proteins react with carbohydrates. What's interesting about AGES is that you can see them. If you've ever seared a steak, browned a loaf of bread, or toasted a marshmallow, you have witnessed first-hand the formation of AGES.

We know that when a person's blood level of AGES is higher, that the markers for inflammation are also higher. Indeed, animal proteins aren't the only source of AGES, but they are a primary source for people who eat the average western diet amount of red meat regularly.

Finally, we have saturated fats, which red meats are high in. Saturated fats create inflammation almost instantly, regardless of the source they're coming from. They also fill your body full of free radicals, creating oxidative stress. There's just nothing good that can be said about saturated fats, especially if you're looking at ways of healing your body, restoring balance, and quieting inflammation.

How Does a Plant-Based Diet Improve Autoimmune Disease?

So, here is where we begin to connect some dots. We don't know what exactly causes autoimmune disorders, but we do know that certain people are in a higher risk group. We also know that inflammation plays a major role in autoimmune disorders, how the disease progresses, and the damage that it causes to the body. Common sense tells us that taking steps towards reducing inflammation and balancing hormones, which can also prevent chronic inflammation, is a good start to not only treating the symptoms of autoimmune disease, and other chronic inflammatory conditions, but also treating the root source of the problem. Can a plant-based diet cure autoimmune disease? There's technically no accepted research that there is ANY cure for autoimmune disease. However, those who adopt a plant-based lifestyle tend to suffer less serious effects of their disease and, in some cases, find that they're able to maintain long-standing remission.

In looking at Rheumatoid arthritis, there is a growing body of research that patients that adopt a plant-based style of eating that includes abundant amounts of nutrients from fruit and vegetables, along with sufficient amounts of fiber (which the standard diet is severely lacking), that they're better able to control their BMI and reduce the pain and inflammation associated with RA. It has been shown that these results can be achieved in as little as four weeks on a low-fat, plant-based diet.

Rheumatoid arthritis is just one example that we're using here. There is both scientific research and plenty of anecdotal evidence to back the claims that a plant-based diet can reduce the severity of other autoimmune disorders, such as lupus, diabetes, and multiple sclerosis.

Eliminating foods that cause inflammation, like dairy, red meat, processed foods, refined sugars, saturated fats, etc., is only one part of the equation. In the case of autoimmune disorders, inflammation is already present. You need to focus not only on reducing inflammation but also doing everything you can to prevent it.

You've heard over and over again that fruits, vegetables, whole grains, and all the nutrients they contain are key to optimal health. One thing that doesn't get mentioned as much, but is so very important, is fiber. The standard American diet doesn't see nearly as much fiber as it should. The average adult needs about 25 to 30 grams of fiber a day. The typical adult consumes maybe half that amount.

Why is fiber so important? Eating a diet that is packed with fiber-rich foods, like fruits, vegetables, and whole grains is protective against many chronic diseases, including cardiovascular disease, diabetes, and arthritis – three health conditions known to be influenced by inflammation.

To understand how fiber affects inflammation, we need to take a detour to discuss the gut biome, which is a fascinating topic on its own. Within your gut is this population of bacteria, both good and bad. They make up their own little microbiome, and in a perfect world, the good bacteria far outnumber the bad guys, and everything runs smoothly. However, our tendency to eat high fat, highly refined foods, along with medications that destroy the natural gut biome, have left things in a less than perfect state for many people.

When your gut biome is out of balance, and the bad guys are overpopulating the place, it isn't just your digestive health that's affected. What happens in your gut affects your health from head to toe, including the effectiveness of your immune system. Dysbiosis, which is a term that's used to describe a microbial imbalance of the gut biome, can lead to a host of chronic diseases, including gut-related autoimmune disorders like Crohn's disease and ulcerative colitis. Dysbiosis has also been linked to obesity and even autism, so you can see that the effects of imbalanced gut bacteria are substantial (Zhang, Li, Gan, Zhou, Xu, & Li, 2015).

In order to have a properly balanced gut biome, you need to first avoid, as much as possible, the things that destroy it. Medications are a common culprit, and this is one reason that we need to be mindful of the overuse of antibiotics and other medications. Illness, stress, lifestyle factors, and the unavoidable process of aging also tend to create less than optimal changes in a healthy gut biome.

The second thing you need to do to support a properly balanced gut biome is to feed the good guys what they need, so they get stronger, multiply, kill off and overcome the army of bad gut bacteria. This is where fiber enters the picture.

As a nutrient, fiber is in a different league. Your body doesn't absorb and synthesize fiber the way that it does other nutrients. For example, when you eat foods rich in vitamin C, your body gets busy putting the vitamin to work. With fiber, it tends to just pass through the body but along the way it does something essential – it feeds all those good gut bacteria and gives them the fuel they need to protect your health. A healthy gut biome equals less inflammation and ultimately less chronic disease.

Fiber isn't the only source of nutrition for a healthy gut biome. Fresh vegetables, especially those that are rich in phytonutrients and antioxidants are great for gut health. So are whole fruits (opt for the actual fruit instead of the juice whenever possible), herbs, healthy fats from sources like avocado or olive oil, and probiotic-rich foods, which include fermented goodness like kombucha, kimchi, and sauerkraut.

What destroys the gut biome, and as a result increases the inflammation related to autoimmune disorders, hormonal imbalance, and other chronic diseases? Primarily non-plant-based foods. Red meats, dairy, poultry, eggs, refined oils, trans fats, processed grains, and foods with added sugars. Notice that there isn't a single plant-based food on the "bad" list. This isn't just a coincidence.

Autoimmune Disorders, Inflammation, Hormonal Imbalances, and the Endocrine System

We've spent quite a bit of time discussing autoimmune disorders in a book that's supposed to be about hormonal health. The reason is that all of this is tied together.

First, let's consider how the hormones, including sex hormones and stress hormones, have a direct effect on immune function. Research has only begun to look at the relationship between these types of hormonal imbalances and the occurrence of autoimmune disease. What we do know is that hormonal imbalance is connected to inflammation, which can increase the severity of autoimmune disorders and possibly supply the spark that leads to full-blown disease.

We know that women are more likely than men to suffer from different types of autoimmune disorders, possibly due to the unique way their body handles hormones. Women are more likely to develop lupus, Hashimoto's thyroiditis, rheumatoid arthritis, and Grave's disease.

When considering the whole of the endocrine system, one gland that is most directly affected by autoimmune disorders is the thyroid. Both Grave's disease and Hashimoto's are inflammatory autoimmune disorders that affect the thyroid and disrupt hormone production.

Grave's disease is an autoimmune disorder where the thyroid produces too much thyroid hormone. When the thyroid is overactive, as is the case with Grave's disease, we call the condition hyperthyroidism. Today, Grave's disease is thought to be the most common cause of hyperthyroidism. This autoimmune disorder affects more women than men, and most commonly occurs between the ages of 20 and 40, however it can develop in both men and women of any age.

When you have Grave's disease, you may notice symptoms related to thyroid hormone imbalance, such as increased fatigue, stress, anxiety, changes in menstrual cycles or sexual function, sensitivity to heat, and sleep disturbances.

As we discussed earlier in this book, the thyroid is one of the main powerhouses of the endocrine system, and achieving a balance in function is essential for overall endocrine health. In the case of Grave's disease, the goal is to help restore proper thyroid function by reducing inflammation. One of the most effective natural methods of achieving this is through diet.

Hashimoto's disease is another autoimmune disorder that affects the thyroid gland. In the case of Hashimoto's disease, the immune system attacks the thyroid and creates chronic inflammation that we call chronic lymphocytic thyroiditis. Hashimoto's disease can eventually lead to reduced thyroid function, which is called hypothyroidism. Hashimoto's disease is thought to be the leading known cause of hypothyroidism. Like Grave's disease, it affects more women than men, however, the average age of onset is slightly older.

Also like Grave's disease, the goal of treating Hashimoto's is to reduce inflammation and restore thyroid function and balance. Some medications are very effective at achieving this goal, and the best course of treatment should be discussed between you and your doctor. However, it's important to not ignore the potential of nutritional healing, and at the very least strive to complement any medications you may be taking by reducing inflammation as much as possible through diet and lifestyle factors.

CHAPTER SUMMARY

In this chapter, we turned the discussion to autoimmune disorders. We know that all autoimmune disorders have one common element - inflammation. Consuming plant-based foods has been shown to be an effective way of soothing inflammation, and thereby slowing or halting the progression of autoimmune diseases. Specifically, we've discussed:

- Traditional medicine, including pharmaceuticals, is often aimed at treating symptoms and not root causes. This is especially true in the case of autoimmune disease
- In autoimmune disorders, an overactive immune system attacks the body's organs and tissues, mistaking them for invasive pathogens

- It's estimated that as many as 23.5 million people suffer from over 80 different types of autoimmune disease
- Each autoimmune disease is unique in how it manifests in the body
- Adopting a plant-based approach to eating can calm inflammation and balance hormones – two key factors in the development and progression of autoimmune disease.

In the next chapter, we're going to discuss what you can do to regain control of your health, balance hormones, and stop inflammation in its tracks. It all starts with learning about plant-based eating and which adaptation of a plant-based diet is best for you.

5

WHAT YOU CAN DO

K nowledge is power, and at this point, you're empowered with an incredible amount of information on how to support your health through a properly functioning endocrine system. I know firsthand that when you're facing such massive changes, that it all starts to feel overwhelming. I personally think this sense of too much all at once is one of the main contributing factors to people giving up on their healthy living goals, and this saddens me deeply.

Life is a journey. You didn't immediately jump from learning the alphabet to landing your first job. There was a process of learning and experience that occurred. You matured, you learned skills, you gained a lifetime of experience along the way that enabled you to succeed when you were finally ready to take that leap into adulthood. It might not be the best analogy but healing the endocrine system is similar in many ways.

You're now starting at this point with a foundation of knowledge. Slowly, over the coming weeks, months, and even years, you're going to learn how to make sustainable changes, your mindset will eventually adapt, and you'll experience improvements in your health – sometimes slowly, other times all at once. Changing the endocrine system is a gradual one, there isn't a quick fix. I want you to experience restored health as quickly as possible but there isn't any rushing in this.

This is why I think it's important to take each person's personality and inclinations into consideration when creating an action plan toward endocrine health. You can go as fast or as slow as you need/want to through this process. The important thing is that you remain consistent. It's not a bad thing to slip up – if you dust yourself off and get right back on your path. Two steps forward and the occasional step back still keeps you moving forward.

What doesn't work for improving endocrine health is inconsistency in your approach. Taking on so much at once, to the point that you're unable to sustain the changes, is worse than making small, manageable changes over a longer time. Take your personality into consideration here. Are you someone that needs to go all in, headfirst, or do you work best when you can achieve success at one or two small changes at a time? Be honest with yourself here because it's important for your overall success.

On this subject, I'm sometimes asked if it's necessary to go all-in on a plant-based diet to fully restore endocrine health. Of course, I'm going to support you going plant-based to the fullest extent you're comfortable with. Whatever level you're comfortable with, adopting plant-based eating habits provides many scientifically proven health benefits.

If the idea of a completely plant-based diet is off-putting to you, consider that there are other ways of including more plant-based foods in your diet, without going 100% all-in.

Plant-Based Diet – All in?

I would absolutely love it if you've found the inspiration in this book to switch to a completely plant-based diet. If you're not comfortable with making the complete switch now, perhaps after a series of slow changes towards a plant-based lifestyle you'll be more comfortable with the idea.

However, plant-based eating isn't the same as plant-only eating. Plant-based means working towards making plant foods the central components of your diet. It doesn't mean that you have to completely eliminate everything that doesn't fit neatly into the plant food category if you're not ready or simply don't want to at this time.

I'd like to take a minute to talk about the different types of plant-based diets, and what makes each of them a little different. Hopefully, you can find one on this list that fits in your comfort zone.

Types of Plant-Based Diets

Semi-Vegetarian – This type of diet consists of mostly plants but allows room for some animal foods, like eggs and dairy. A semi-vegetarian diet would also include the occasional serving of animal proteins, like seafood or non-red meats. I say non-red meat here because red meat has been shown to increase the risk of heart disease and early morbidity (Northwestern University, 2020). There is also enough research to begin implicating red meat in an increased risk of certain types of cancers. If you choose a semi-vegetarian lifestyle, eat animal proteins sparingly, and make sure they're lean and unprocessed.

Pescatarian – A pescatarian diet is one that is primarily vegetarian but includes fish and seafood as sources of non-plant-based protein. A pescatarian diet is more heart-healthy than a non-vegetarian diet, and it's also rich in healthy fats. There are a few things to keep in mind when choosing a pescatarian lifestyle. The first is to still keep plant-based foods at the center of your diet. Too much fish and seafood can have negative health consequences, especially depending on the type of fish and how it was raised/farmed. Also, be mindful when preparing fish and seafood. Avoid frying, tons of butter, and heavy sauces.

Vegetarian – Following a vegetarian diet means you do not consume animal proteins, including meat, poultry, wild game, fish, seafood, or any foods that are the by-products of the animals raised for slaughter – such as lard or tallow. There are different types of vegetarianism. Some, like lacto-ovo vegetarians, include animal foods that aren't the result of a slaughtered animal, like eggs, dairy, and honey.

Vegan – A vegan diet is one that excludes all foods that can be traced back to an animal source. This includes all meat, eggs, dairy, honey, whey, etc. A class of veganism called ethical vegans also avoid non-food products that are made from animals, such as leather shoes, cosmetics that include animal-based ingredients, and lanolin. What's important to remember when choosing a vegan diet is that just because it doesn't contain animal products doesn't mean it's healthy. Oreos are considered vegan but are far from healthy or plant-based.

Benefits of Plant-Based Diets

Alright, we've done a lot of talking about how a plant-based diet is beneficial for your endocrine system and autoimmune health. If you're like me, you don't want to read through this entire book every time you need a refresher or a little inspiration to keep moving toward a plant-based lifestyle. Here is a quick reference list of some of the top benefits of plant-based diets.

- *Weight-management* – Most people find that weight loss occurs naturally when switching to a plant-based diet and that weight maintenance is achieved with little effort. If you're someone who needs to gain weight or can't afford to lose weight, make sure you include extra healthy fats and calorically dense plant-based foods like avocados and nuts.

- *Reduced Inflammation* – Adopting a plant-based diet is one of the quickest ways to reduce inflammation in your body. Chronic inflammation is a precursor to almost all of today's chronic health conditions, and it's disruptive to endocrine function. Less chronic inflammation in your body leads to improved longevity.

- *Cardiovascular Health* – Along with less inflammation, you also benefit from improved cardiovascular health when you adopt a plant-based lifestyle. All those saturated fats, processed sugars, and inflammation-causing foods are bad for your ticker.

- *Protection Against Diabetes* – Diabetes is an inflammatory disease, and once you begin to reduce the inflammation in your body through a plant-based diet, you begin offering yourself more protection against developing the disease. If you have already been diagnosed with type II diabetes, adopting a plant-based diet can help control your disease.

- *Longer Life Expectancy* – Plant-based diets don't contribute to the onset of chronic health conditions in the way that the standard American diet does. It makes sense that less disease equals a lower mortality risk by preventable health-related causes. There have also been numerous studies to back up the theory that adopting a plant-based diet can increase life expectancy, at least into the ninth decade (GE).

- *Sharper Mind* – We're going to circle back around to inflammation yet again. Inflammation is a central factor in cognitive decline as we age. There is interesting research occurring that looks at the effect of plant-based diets on slowing the progression of Alzheimer's. A plant-based diet also promotes sharper focus and concentration while doing everyday tasks. Who knows, start eating more plants and your boss might be so impressed with your enhanced performance that they offer you that long-deserved raise.

- *Endocrine Health* – Honestly, I could go on all day about the positive effects of a plant-based diet, but our main focus here really is endocrine health. Adopting a plant-based diet is one of the single most effective steps you can take toward restoring hormonal balance and improving endocrine function

First Steps to Embracing a Plant-Based Lifestyle

In my personal experience, it's easy to round up the motivation for change. You want to feel better, look better, be healthier, live longer, and have the energy to fully embrace the life you're living. I love seeing people excited about making these positive changes in their lives. I also know that being excited about something and putting it into practice are two very different things. The execution is often more difficult than planning.

Once you've decided to make changes in your life to balance and heal your endocrine system, the focus turns to "how". How do you make these changes, while doing it in a way that ensures this is a true lifestyle change, and not just passing interest? If you were sitting in front of me right now, we could talk about how to implement these changes in your life, the challenges you might face, and how to overcome them.

Since we don't have the luxury of an intimate conversation around changing your life for the better, I can offer a few tips that I think work well for the majority of people. I know we all have unique circumstances that can make parts of this more difficult. My goal here is to provide you with enough tools that you can overcome challenges and opposition, regardless of where it's coming from.

This brings me to a point that isn't always easy to talk about, but I feel it needs to be brought up. The challenges you might face as you're changing your lifestyle and improving your health don't always come from where you might expect. You might find that as you begin making positive changes that some people in your life might react in a way that feels negative. I truly hope that you're surrounded by people who are supportive but it's good to be aware of the possibility that not everyone will be.

As you begin making these changes, the people around you are going to see noticeable changes. These changes might include the way you look but also your general demeanor as you gain energy and suffer less from chronic health issues. You're transforming into a new version of yourself and that can be difficult for some people to accept, even when they know these changes are for the best.

You might also have people who give you a bit of backlash for moving towards a plant-based diet, even if you don't go completely all in. I read an interesting study that looked at the perception of veganism, and how the societal stigma associated with it could explain the barrier some meat-eaters feel about making a complete switch to plant-based eating (Rosenfeld & Tomiyama, 2019).

I feel like the same stigma sometimes holds true for people who make even a partial switch, to just reduce the number of animal products they consume. I think this negative response stems from a mixture of a lack of nutritional knowledge, their personal history of food, and that by making these types of changes you're criticizing their lifestyle – even if you aren't doing so directly.

These negative reactions don't often stem from a place of malice but rather a place of misunderstanding. If you encounter these types of reactions, you might feel defensive or discouraged. I want to suggest that your response be gentle and informative. Some people will truly want to learn why you're making these changes, but they don't want to feel judged themselves. Others will remain skeptical no matter what. It's best to not give too much of your energy to these types.

If someone seems to be truly toxic, I hope that you can find a way to limit contact with this person in your life. Continue to remind yourself that this is about your health and how you feel in this one body you're given.

Okay, now that we've said that let's move on to some of the most effective tips for the beginning stages of changing your diet and embracing a healthier lifestyle.

Change Your Mindset About Meat and Dairy

This is something that many people will find incredibly hard. If you've been eating the standard American diet, meat and dairy have probably been mealtime staples your entire life. We tend to form very strong emotional connections to food. Certain foods become part of our traditions and part of our personal stories. It's normal at first to feel like you're giving up a part of yourself by changing your eating habits.

For instance, if you grew up celebrating Thanksgiving with a traditional meal, it might be unthinkable to imagine the holiday without a huge turkey taking up the center of the table. Maybe it's a simple routine like going out for burgers with friends or family every Friday to celebrate the end of the week. If you've eaten meat and dairy your entire life, chances are you have at least a few fond memories built around these foods.

First, as we discussed just a bit ago, you don't have to give up these foods completely. I would make the case that if you do want to keep these types of foods in your life, eating them sparingly or only on holidays or special occasions is the perfect balance of holding onto your history with food while also making major strides in rebuilding your health.

Still, the fact remains that you can't continue to keep eating like you have and achieve the changes in your health that you're looking for. So, you have to make changes and for you, that might mean changing how you think about meat and its role in your diet.

If you're not keen on the idea of giving up meat entirely, you might start by thinking differently about how you incorporate meat and other animal products into your meals. Instead of thinking of meat as the main component of your meals, think of it as a garnish. Simple switches like adding a bit of meat to a sauce or sprinkling shredded chicken on a veggie taco. Start getting in the mindset that meat doesn't need to be the star of the show at every meal.

One concern that I hear repeatedly about eliminating or reducing meat consumption is the idea that you need more protein than you can consume on a plant-based diet. First, there are so many sources of plant-based protein, that if you're eating a well-rounded diet, this really shouldn't be a concern.

You don't need as much protein as you think you do. Protein is essential but our society is a little protein obsessed right now. Exactly how much protein you should consume each day depends on factors like your age, weight, and activity level.

Generally speaking, you're going to want to take in about 10-30% (with the higher end of this spectrum being for people who are physically active and build muscle) of your body weight in protein. You can also use the standard calculation of your weight in kilograms and multiply it by .80 to determine how many grams you need.

The standard American diet, which typically contains meat at nearly every meal, is possibly too high in protein. Your body has a max amount of protein that it can process and utilize each day. When someone exceeds this amount for an extended duration of time, they put their body at risk of serious health consequences, including osteoporosis, liver or kidney disease, and an increased risk of certain cancers. One study looked at a group of women who consumed 5 servings of red meat per week and compared them to women who consumed less than one ounce per week. Their findings revealed that women with higher protein levels suffered more bone fractures (Delimaris, 2019). When it comes to protein, more isn't always better.

There's this idea that protein can only come from animal sources. If you're eating a variety of foods on a plant-based diet that includes foods like lentils, black beans, tofu, quinoa, chickpeas, hemp seeds, and nuts, you're not going to be lacking in protein. In fact, you'll likely end up with the perfect amount, without even giving it much thought.

Amp Up Your Veggie Intake

Eating more vegetables every day can be challenging at first, especially if you usually reach for a prepacked, processed option come snack time. Getting used to eating more vegetables daily is one of those things you just have to jump in and start doing in order for it to feel like a more normal part of your routine. Once you get more accustomed to the taste and texture of a variety of vegetables, reaching for them first becomes second nature.

I have a few strategies that I encourage my clients to use when amping up their veggie intake. The first is to replace any processed or animal-based foods that you snack on with vegetables instead. Instead of chips and dip, reach for cut veggies and salsa or hummus. Instead of the gooey queso with your tortilla chips, substitute in guacamole and maybe snack on carrots sticks instead of fried chips.

Buying vegetables that you can prepare ahead of time for easy snacking or to quickly add to a meal is key to success in this area. The next time you go grocery shopping, have a goal of trying at least two new snackable vegetables. By snackable, I mean anything delicious when eaten raw. Snow peas, broccoli, shaved Brussels sprouts, sliced bell peppers of every color…. you get the picture. In the produce section, you're sure to find a few favorites and new things to try. Use this transitional time as a chance to try new things and expand your horizons.

Shifting the focus of your meals from animal products to vegetables is another way to make your transition easier. Try making it a goal to fill half your plate with vegetables at both lunch and dinner. Also, don't get stuck in a color rut. Enjoying a colorful variety of foods will help ensure you're getting optimal nutrition from your food.

Now is also a good time to rethink how you eat vegetables. For some people, their only experience with vegetables have been boiled, overcooked, mushy vegetables served to them as a child. Others might think that salads are the only real way to eat vegetables and that can easily get boring. Expand your cooking repertoire here. There are so many incredible ways to eat vegetables that once you master a few techniques, you're less likely to miss and crave all the extra animal protein in your diet.

Don't Neglect Fiber

This is a big one. When working with my clients, I really try to drive this one home. Fiber plays such a central role in your health. We tend to think of fiber as being important only to gut health but as we're learning, gut health has a tremendous impact on our overall state of wellbeing, including hormonal health.

When you consume enough dietary fiber, you're working to protect yourself against serious chronic health concerns, including hormone-related conditions. Adequate fiber intake can offer protection against digestive disorders, heart disease, diabetes, obesity, hypertension, stroke, and some cancers.

Fiber does other amazing things, too. Adequate fiber intake can help you feel more satiated with each meal, fend off cravings for unhealthy food during the day, and stabilize your blood glucose levels, which can provide you with more stamina and focus during the day. It really is great stuff.

What I've found, and there's research to back me up on this, is that the issue isn't that people don't understand the importance of fiber in their diets. It's that there are misconceptions about the best sources of fiber, coupled with the fact that many people think they consume more than they do.

When comparing studies on the subject, about two-thirds of people believe they consume adequate amounts of fiber daily. However, when looking at actual dietary intake, only about 5% of us are getting enough (Quagliani & Felt-Gunderson). This is an incredibly stark contrast and leads one to wonder where the difference in what we do vs what we think we're doing is coming from.

I'm going to pinpoint two major contributors here, although I'm sure there are others. The first is the fad diet trends that lead you to believe you need less fiber in your diet than you actually do. The typical person needs to consume in the range of 25-30 grams of fiber per day. The average person consumes about half of that. Diets that promote animal-based foods or eliminate major sources of wholesome dietary fiber, such as Keto and Paleo type plans, simply don't put enough emphasis on the fiber intake that's necessary to support your health.

The second culprit I want to shine a light on here is the food industry and marketing. It amazes me (and not in a good way) when I go to a store, pick up a box of "high-fiber" cereal, and read the label only to find that it's dismally low in fiber. It might be high in fiber compared to other cereal options but relying on one or two packaged products for your daily fiber intake is going to leave you with a serious deficit.

In contrast, you're going to find many different rich sources of fiber with plant-based foods. A cup of lentils and some broccoli in one meal can bring you up to 20 grams of fiber. Add in some raspberries, a serving of whole grains, and a handful of nuts throughout the day, and you've easily reached the recommended 25-30 grams.

Start Your Day with Whole Grains

Returning to the point we just discussed about getting enough fiber, the longer into the day you wait to add in fiber, the more difficult it becomes to reach the suggested intake. If you've gone all day, barely consuming any fiber at all, trying to stuff in 25 grams at dinner is going to be an uncomfortable experience.

I always suggest to my clients that they start their day with whole grains. Not only does this set you off on a great start for meeting your daily fiber requirements, but whole grains are also nutritious, filling, and will help keep your blood sugar and hormone levels in check during the first part of your day. Once you get into this habit, you might even find that you don't need so much coffee to get your engine revving.

I'm talking about starting your day with real whole grains here, like the breakfast staple of oatmeal. Not the kind in little packages with that powdered, sugary flavor mix but steel-cut oats that you enhance yourself with spices, fruit, nuts, and maybe a little bit of honey. If you're gluten-sensitive or gluten intolerant, gluten-free grains like quinoa, amaranth, buckwheat, and sorghum are all nutritious, filling whole grains that are perfect for starting your day.

Whole grains provide the ideal nutritional canvas to start your day. They're rich in B vitamins, minerals, protein, antioxidants, and plant compounds that are key in fighting disease.

Have a plan to make your morning grains more interesting. Adding some fruit or nuts is a great way to boost nutritional value even higher. Plant-based kinds of milk are great for cooking grains in or adding to them if you like cold cereal. Spices are also your friend, so try experimenting with cinnamon, nutmeg, ginger, turmeric, cloves, allspice.... get creative.

Don't Overwhelm Yourself

There are a couple of different schools of thought about how to best begin a drastic dietary change like the one I'm suggesting to support your hormonal health. You know yourself better than anyone else, so I ask you to be honest with yourself about how to best make this transition.

Some people are most likely to achieve long-term success with an all or nothing approach. They completely switch their diets and lifestyle overnight, going all in. If you're someone who works best with this type of structure, I want you to at least be prepared for the possibility that you may have some short-term unpleasantness as your body detoxes, which we'll talk about more in just a bit. You might also have a bit of digestive upset if you suddenly go from a low fiber to a high fiber diet. If you suddenly switch from a diet full of processed foods to one full of fruits, vegetables, and grains, your body will go through a period of adjustment.

If you're someone who acclimates best to big changes by taking them one step at a time, I want to encourage you to not overwhelm yourself. This is a lifelong journey you're taking, and while I want to see you achieve healthy results as quickly as possible, I also want these changes to be sustainable for you.

One way to start, and this works especially well if you have others in your household who might be resistant to the idea of a plant-based lifestyle, is to begin by cooking one meal each week that is completely free of animal protein and dairy. Build this meal with hearty, filling, flavorful ingredients that can be adapted to a range of taste preferences. Start with a selection from the rainbow of beans available, a whole grain, and mountains of vegetables that will fill you up, add texture, and help you to not feel "deprived". If you love the texture of meat, mushrooms have a great meaty consistency to them when cooked.

Once you've mastered one meal a week, try going an entire day eating no animal protein or dairy. This approach gives you time to experiment with new foods, flavors, and recipes – and it also gives your body time to adjust to the changes.

You can probably see where I'm going next with this but once you feel comfortable with an entire meat/dairy-free day, build that into two days, then three. If you want to go completely plant-based, keep at it until you get there. If you've decided you still want to allow a small amount of meat/dairy in your diet, aim to eat those types of foods only one to two days a week, and keep portions small.

Recreate Mealtime

So many of us in this society have been brought up thinking that a meal consisted of meat, bread or maybe pasta, a starchy vegetable like potatoes or corn, and maybe a small salad on the side is a healthy meal. Unfortunately, this is far from the truth. This type of diet doesn't offer the degree of nutritional density that you need to be the healthiest version of yourself, and it doesn't support hormonal health.

Recreating mealtime is an important step to starting and staying the course in changing your dietary lifestyle. One of my favorite things, and something I regularly suggest to my clients, is to build an entire meal where the salad is the centerpiece and not the side dish. I love this because it's so versatile and you can create endless variations of it. You can also use whatever you happen to have on hand, which saves you a trip to the grocery store and keeps the grocery budget in check.

Start with a big bowl full of your favorite greens or try a new one. Spinach, romaine, and Bibb lettuce make an excellent salad base, and these greens are high in nutritional density. Red leafy greens are also great, as are heartier greens like kale.

Next, pile on anything you like. Don't be bashful here, this isn't your wimpy side salad. Add in fresh herbs for a punch of flavor, a variety of vegetables, beans, or tofu for added protein and fiber, nuts, seeds, fruits.... seriously, go crazy.

Have a sweet tooth that loves to be satisfied with a decadent dessert? I'm not going to suggest you go out for a hot fudge sundae but there's no reason you can't indulge your craving for something sweet after a meal. The only difference is that fruit should be the centerpiece.

Honestly, there just aren't many things more delicious than a bowl full of ripe, sweet berries on their own. Sliced fresh fruit, arranged beautifully on a plate is decadent on its own. You can also cook fruits, while maybe adding a bit of spice, to release all the natural sweet juices.

Finally, work on adding in more healthy fats into your diet. Of course, you don't want to go overboard with any type of fat because they're so calorically dense that you don't want to over-consume. However, healthy, plant-based fats like olive oil, avocado oil, and walnut oil are perfect for sprinkling over your foods in small amounts. You can also skip the oil and head to the source by slicing up an avocado and olives or enjoying a small handful of nuts. These types of fats are beneficial to your endocrine system and your cardiovascular health.

Detox Period

If you read blogs about the plant-based lifestyle or visit forums and groups that offer advice and support to people who are transitioning toward a more plant-forward way of eating, you'll read countless stories from people who say their lives have completely changed with their diet. They feel great, have incredible energy, amazing clarity, and focus, and many of their chronic health issues have just up and left the room.

There are so many incredible benefits to embracing this style of eating, and a healthier lifestyle in general. Still, I don't want to brush over the fact that, for most people, the body goes through a period of adjustment as you make these changes. Consider that so many of the foods included in the standard American diet are loaded with salt, sugars, preservatives, and processed ingredients. Your body has become accustomed to processing these types of foods daily. There is an inevitable detox period that occurs as your diet shifts to support your hormonal health.

Depending on how fast or slow you make these changes, you might experience a few days of detox symptoms or a couple of weeks. You need to understand during this time that the process you're going through isn't one that should happen magically overnight. Resetting your hormonal balance is something that's going to take time. If plowing in headfirst is too challenging for you, especially if you're experiencing more severe symptoms of withdrawal, it's okay to slow down and do this at a pace that feels right for your body.

Some people experience what you might call a detox flu when they change their dietary lifestyle. You might experience mild symptoms such as headaches, fatigue, lack of concentration, and a general feeling of blah for a couple of days. This is a normal process as your body resets itself. I promise it won't last forever and there are some simple things you can do to offer relief during the detox period.

- Get plenty of rest. This isn't the time to skimp on getting adequate sleep.
- Drink lots of hydrating fluids. Coffee, caffeinated teas, and soft drinks are the answer to keep you going through this.
- Don't skip meals. This is important. Eating more of a plant-based diet probably means that you're consuming fewer calories than you were. It's important to not let your caloric intake tank too low.
- Give yourself space. You might find you're a little irritable for a couple of days. Give yourself some space and quiet.
- Don't expect too much of yourself. You don't have to switch your diet completely in one day. You don't have

to give up everything at once. You don't have to jump into a fitness routine on the same day you start making changes in your diet. Respect your body and the process by giving yourself adequate time to adjust.

- Know this is your journey and yours alone. If you're making these changes with a buddy (which is a great idea, by the way) what you experience and feel might be very different. This isn't a competition or a place for judgment. Each of our bodies is unique.
- Maintain a food log and be specific. Record what you eat, what time you eat it, how you feel, and anything you notice throughout the day. This will help you find dietary solutions to your health issues and provide inspiration as you begin to see positive changes.

The extent of dietary changes that any one person needs to make varies widely depending on the severity of their hormonal imbalance and the symptoms they're experiencing. This is, of course, going to affect your detox period.

The ultimate goal here is to remove all processed foods, refined sugars, dairy products, and gluten. I know we haven't talked that much about gluten because we've been focused more on animal-based foods. It's estimated that about 1% of people in the United States are living with Celiac disease. More common, however, is gluten sensitivity, which is thought to affect at least 6% of the US population (Igbinedion, Ansari, Vasikaran, Gavins, Jordan, Boktor, ... & Alexander, 2017).

Keep in mind that these are mostly people with pronounced symptoms of intolerance. While numbers are difficult to come by, there is plenty of anecdotal evidence to suggest that the number of people affected by gluten sensitivities, especially regarding inflammation and hormonal response, is significantly higher

So, if you're feeling overwhelmed right now, work to eliminate the big four that I just mentioned – processed foods (yes, all of them), refined sugars, dairy products, and gluten. Do them one at a time if you're finding it a challenge. Deciding to eat a certain way is one thing. Knowing how to grocery shop and preparing meals that you're going to enjoy, without too much fuss every single day, is quite another. Work at your own pace, just make sure you keep working. After the initial detox period, as your endocrine system begins to restore balance, you're going to start seeing and feeling incredible changes.

4 STEPS TO AUTOIMMUNE IMPROVEMENT

At this point, I hope that you're excited, or at least encouraged, to begin making some dietary and lifestyle changes that will rebuild and support your hormonal health. A major component of this is working towards autoimmune improvement. I've broken down the path to autoimmune improvement into 4 steps to help you better understand the process.

Step 1: Eliminate Foods with the Most Potential for Reactions

This first step is the foundation of this book. The foods we consume have such a profound effect on our health, often in ways, we're completely unaware of. This single step of eliminating foods with the most potential for reactions is where you're going to see the most significant gains. This step is also necessary to achieve before moving onto the next ones.

If you're taking medications for hormonal or autoimmune health conditions, please don't stop without first discussing the decision with a health care provider. There are circumstances in which medications are essential in treating disease. But I also have a firm belief in the body's ability to restore balance when we provide it with the nutrition that it needs and eliminate the things that make it difficult for the body to perform optimally.

Medications often treat the symptoms, which is fine when you're looking for relief this minute. I want you to experience more than just relief. My wish is for you to experience true healing and a restoration of balance.

So, to review. Start by cutting out the foods that promote inflammation and hormonal imbalance. These include processed foods, refined sugars, dairy, gluten, and animal protein – especially red meat.

Step 2: Reduce Inflammation

Step 2 is the natural consequence of step 1 but there are other things you can be doing to further reduce chronic inflammation that can sabotage your health, ignite flares in your autoimmune disease, and disrupt hormonal harmony.

Reducing inflammation, outside of dietary, involves making yourself a priority. Take time each day to de-stress and relax. This helps calm hormonal surges that lead to inflammation. Regular exercise is also a great tool for keeping inflammation at bay – just make sure you honor your body and don't push too hard if you have injuries, mobility concerns, or health issues that affect how strenuously you should exercise.

Step 3: Create a Healthy Gut Environment

Plant-focused diets are naturally high in fiber, which is great for your gut environment. Fiber from a plant-based diet feeds all the good bacteria in your gut, which help to keep the endocrine system functioning properly, balance hormones, and reduce inflammation. A diet that's high in fiber increases these little things called short-chain fatty acids. Short-chain fatty acids are known to enhance intestinal function and boost the immune system, but in a way that doesn't present a risk to those who suffer from autoimmune disease.

To create and maintain a healthy gut environment, aim to meet the daily fiber intake recommendations of 25-30 grams. Include prebiotic and probiotic foods to give all that good bacteria a little boost and avoid foods that can damage gut flora – like those that are high in processed sugars and other ingredients that promote inflammation.

Step 4: Promote Immune Health

Whether your immune system is underactive or overactive, as is the case with autoimmune disease, doing whatever you can to promote immune health is essential to your overall well-being, endocrine health, and managing autoimmune disorders.

As you begin to make changes in your diet and lifestyle, improved immune health is a natural consequence. Still, you want to keep immune health in mind as you make decisions about how you're going to nourish, care for, and respect your body.

Inflammation is a precursor to many types of diseases. If you can get to the point where inflammation is under control, then you've accomplished overcoming one of the biggest obstacles in achieving optimal immune function. In my practice, I've worked with clients who have experienced significant gains in the management of their autoimmune conditions, simply by choosing foods that calm inflammation and nourish the body, rather than those that put even more stress on the immune system.

Diet is important for promoting immune health, but the approach should also be holistic. Respect your body, treat yourself with kindness, and learn to permit yourself to make your physical and mental health a priority. Eliminate stressful situations as much as possible, and work toward developing coping strategies for those you can't control. Make a little time for yourself each day to keep stress at a baseline minimum.

CHAPTER SUMMARY

In this chapter, we looked at the value of plant-based eating and how it can work in your life. Plant-based diets offer a ton of healthy benefits, but you don't have to go 100% plant-based to see improvements. Specifically, we've discussed:

- Plant-based diets have health benefits including, hormonal balance, reduced inflammation, weight loss, improve cardiovascular health, and so much more
- Plant-based eating isn't plant-only eating - you can do this in the way that works best for you
- Take it easy on yourself as you transition toward incorporating more plant-based foods in your diet, and expect a detox period where you might not feel so great
- Take it step by step to improve hormonal balance and improve autoimmune symptoms.

In the next chapter, we celebrate getting to the point where you're ready to make these changes happen. It takes commitment but you're going to be stronger and healthier for it.

6

A LIFE THAT WILL LAST

The dietary changes that we've discussed making in this book are life-altering in so many ways. When you've been living with the symptoms of endocrine dysfunction, it can be difficult to believe that you'll ever regain your health and feel as good as you once did. The changes I'm outlining in this book aren't easy but when you commit to them, you are taking powerful steps to achieve balanced hormonal function and improved health.

Consistent, sustainable results are key to maintaining proper hormonal function throughout your life. I know how frustrating it is to jump in, make the changes, and experience positive results – only to backtrack later and lose the ground you gained. Life happens, which is why I truly want to set you up with a sustainable plan, one that you can adapt to and fit easily into your life, regardless of what's happening around you.

Making any type of sustainable, major dietary change is an ongoing, evolving process. You're going to build upon the knowledge you have today, which means you might make different dietary decisions in the future. It's too difficult, or even impossible, to absorb all this information at once. So, you take it in, in manageable amounts, and make changes as you go. As we know better, we do better.

You're currently at a pinnacle point on your journey to hormonal wellness. Right now, you are armed with a strong foundation of knowledge that includes a basic understanding of what the endocrine system is, how it functions, and the significant role it plays in your overall health. You've also learned how dietary choices can affect hormones, endocrine function, and everything that's connected with it.

Now, the ball is in your court to commit yourself. A commitment to make the changes and stick to them as your health evolves along this journey. Making real changes in your health requires real dedication, and most importantly, consistency.

Short Term Results Lead to Long Term Progress

I think one of the most difficult aspects of making any type of life-altering change is that you don't always see or feel the results right away. You're there, putting in the work every day, yet the cumulative effects of your actions take time to manifest. I've seen this time and again with people who want to lose weight or change to a more heart-healthy diet. Those types of changes do take time, just like many of the changes you want to achieve by changing your diet to support your hormonal health.

Waiting for results can feel like torture but there's something that you need to know. The very minute you begin making changes in your diet and lifestyle, positive changes begin to occur in your body as well. Think of these first days and weeks as planting a seed. When planting a garden, you don't expect it to sprout overnight but you know each time you water the soil, you're doing something to actively encourage growth. This is what's happening in your body.

Every time you choose a plant-based, anti-inflammatory food over a standard American diet option, you're doing something to prevent your health issues from getting worse while building towards healthier endocrine function. You can't see or feel the results in those first few days, but you know something is sprouting.

After a few days, you begin to feel a little better. You have more energy, the brain fog begins to lift, your mood improves, and maybe you notice less pain from inflammation. This is like the sprout that first erupts from the soil. It's not the end result but it's exactly what you need as confirmation that you're doing the right thing. Over time, your body is like that plant that grows, becoming stronger with each day until it finally blooms.

My point here is that even the small things you do today lead to long term results. I'm continually looking at research on this subject and I'm still always amazed at how quick and profound the effects are of switching to a plant-based diet. Short term studies, some covering just 1-3 months, show noticeable gains in health on multiple levels, from improved mental clarity to enhanced immune function, reduced inflammation, and hormonal balance.

Small gains, when continually achieved over time, lead to significant changes in your health. While you can switch your diet for a short time and experience positive results, the true benefits occur when the effects of these changes are compounded over time.

You Can Do It!

I've been trying to drive home the point here that changes don't happen overnight, especially when considering the complexities of the endocrine system. Your body needs to take in all these nutrients, detox itself from the processed and animal-based foods you've been eating for years. It took time for your body to reach the state that it's currently in, and it will take time to reverse these changes.

If improving your health is important to you, staying on course is non-negotiable. Are these changes difficult? For many, yes. Will there be times you feel like giving up and reverting to your old dietary habits? We're talking about a lifetime here, and yes there will be challenges. You are strong enough to withstand them because your health is important to you.

I've made a point of referring to these changes as a dietary life-style, rather than just calling it a diet. The word diet is full of emotional connotations for so many people. It also alludes to short term changes to reach one specific result. This isn't what we want here.

A bit of research published some time ago by The American Journal of Clinical Nutrition mentioned that about 20% of people who attempted to follow a diet for weight loss purposes succeeded at doing so long term (Wing & Phelan, 2005). Other more recent bodies of research support similar numbers, although success rates tend to flux just a bit based on what type of fad diet was popular at the point of research. I use numbers targeted at dieting for weight loss because numbers of people who succeed in "diets" for other health care reasons are difficult to find. The point here is that only about a fifth of people will adhere to a diet long-term but what if the changes you make aren't a diet, but lifestyle adaptations instead?

I think an important part of succeeding in dietary changes long term is accepting that you're human. If you've been eating animal products your entire life, these changes will be difficult. If you're accustomed to meat or dairy at every meal, you might feel unsatisfied, cheated, or even resentful that your health has to lead you to the point where you need to give up some of your favorite things. Spending time with people who don't follow the same dietary principles as you are challenging, especially on occasions centered around food. You might feel envy, anger, depression, and anxiety over your health and the changes you're making.

All of this is normal and experiencing any of it doesn't mean you're not cut out for the journey ahead of you. Please keep in mind that you can make these changes at the pace that feels most comfortable to you unless you have a medical condition that requires more urgent action. You can allow yourself to feel a range of emotions. I encourage you to journal your emotional journey through this process, as well as your physical one. You're also going to grow stronger and feel more confident in yourself as you stick to your path, even when you slip a little and need to get back up.

You're setting the foundation for a lifetime of change and improved health. Give yourself grace and encouragement. This is a lifetime goal, not a quick race to the finish line.

How Long Before You Start Noticing Real Changes in Your Health?

Here's the big question. How much time do you need to invest in these lifestyle and dietary changes before you start feeling better and achieving noticeable results?

For most people, the real magic starts happening around the 2-week mark. That said, each person is different, as are the health issues they're facing. Some people begin to feel some type of relief from symptoms like inflammation or mental fog almost immediately. Others will need to stick to it a little longer before they start noticing improvements.

When the changes do start kicking in, they're not going to go unnoticed. One of the first places you might notice the effects of a plant-based diet is in the level of inflammation you experience. Those who follow a plant-based diet for at least 2 months almost all report experiencing less inflammation than when they were consuming a diet that contained more animal products, and as a result, more saturated fats. This alone is mostly anecdotal evidence but we also know that a diet that focuses more on plant-based foods results in fewer markers for inflammation, like C-reactive protein.

When you begin to experience these changes in how you feel, know that it isn't all in your mind. You're doing incredible work, that's sometimes challenging. The results are well-deserved and not a fluke.

Feeling Satisfied with Nutritional Balance

Earlier, we briefly touched on the protein factor of a plant-based diet. I want to reiterate that if you're eating a variety of plant-based foods, including grains, nuts, legumes, and vegetables, that you're almost guaranteed to meet the daily requirements for protein with little issue. If you're physically active, actively working on building muscle, or have other special dietary needs, you might need to pay a little bit more attention to make sure you're loading plenty of plant-based protein on your plates. Women who are pregnant also need to be extra diligent about protein since it can affect blood supply and fetal development.

But protein isn't just a dietary need. For many, it offers a feeling of fullness, satiety, and makes a meal feel more complete. If you're someone who has eaten large amounts of protein-rich animal foods, adding in a little extra plant-based protein will likely make the transition easier for you.

When I work with my clients, I make a point of going over the most readily available plant-based sources of protein. It's easy to go wild, stuffing your grocery cart with all the colorful fruits and vegetables from the protein section but people are often confused about exactly where to get protein. Here are a few of my favorite high-protein, plant-based foods.

Soy

Soy-based products like tofu, tempeh, and edamame are among the highest protein plant-based foods. Some years back, soy got a bit of a bad reputation as being a hormone disruptor and possibly being implicated in a higher incidence of hormone-related cancers. Since then, new research has suggested that the old studies don't hold much weight. However, if you've had hormone-related cancer or are at a higher risk, you should speak with a knowledgeable health practitioner about the role of phytoestrogens in your diet.

For the rest of you, soy-based products are an excellent protein alternative to animal meats. A ½ cup of firm tofu contains 10g of protein, and tempeh contains about 50% more. Mix it up and include various types of tofu, tempeh, and delicious edamame. Soy products are also great for replacing the mouthfeel that comes with animal proteins.

Lentils, Chickpeas, and All Sorts of Beans

This category of plant-based foods contains some of the most nutrient-dense sources of protein you can find. Lentils, both red and green, are packed with plenty of protein (more than 8.5 grams per ½ cup), along with lots of fiber, potassium, and iron. Chickpeas (hummus, yum) and other beans aren't far behind on the protein or nutrition scale. What is great about this group of high-protein foods is their versatility. They can be the star of the dish or a compliment, and they blend into just about every imaginable style of cuisine.

Almonds

Most nuts are excellent sources of protein, but almonds are a favorite. First, they're delicious raw, so you don't need extra oil or salt to fully enjoy them. Second, they have more than 16 grams of protein per half-cup. Third, they're rich in vitamin E, which is a powerful antioxidant. A handful of almonds and you're on your way to filling your protein requirement and protecting your body against oxidative stress. A note of caution

– almonds are calorically dense and satisfying. It can be hard to stop at a single handful, but you also don't want to overdo it.

Nuts and Seeds

I listed almonds separately because of their high protein content but most nuts and seeds fall into the high-protein category, and there are just too many to list separately. Nuts and seeds are also a good source of healthy fats and fiber. Here are a few of my favorite high-protein nuts and seeds to add to salads, smoothies, cereal, practically any meal, or to enjoy as a snack.

- Peanuts
- Pistachios
- Walnuts
- Cashews
- Hemp seeds
- Chia seeds
- Sunflower seeds
- Flax seeds
- Pumpkin seeds

Spirulina

Ever looked at a green smoothie and wondered what was in it? Well, it could be some type of delicious leafy, dark green like spinach or kale, but it also could be something called spirulina. Spirulina is a nutrient-rich algae that's also high in protein. Just 2 tablespoons contain about 8 grams of protein. Turned off by the idea of algae? Don't be. You can sprinkle spirulina largely unnoticed over salads, into soups, beverages, or add it to your favorite smoothie blend.

High Protein Grains

We tend to think of grains as providing energy from carbohydrates more than we think of them as being a source of protein. However, you might be surprised to know that some grains are nearly as high in protein as beans, nuts, and seeds. Kamut, teff, spelt, amaranth, and quinoa all hover near 9-10grams of protein per cup. Enjoy them cooked with a sprinkling of nuts or seeds for breakfast, or as a later meal combined with beans and a bounty of vegetables. Either way, you're not going to be lacking for protein.

High Protein Vegetables

Yes, vegetables can have protein, too. Not as much as a cup full of beans, tofu, or grains but definitely enough to help you feel satiated and make a nice contribution to meeting your daily protein requirement. Green peas, spinach, asparagus, corn, mushrooms, broccoli, artichokes, and brussels sprouts all contain a few grams of protein per serving and offer so much more from a nutritional perspective.

Treating Disease without Medication

Now, I'd like to address a subject that is quite sensitive to many people out there. I want to talk about your body's innate ability to heal itself when provided with proper nutrition that eliminates known inflammation and autoimmune triggers, such as red meat and other animal products. This is a bit of a touchy subject because there are some less than credible "experts" out there claiming that medication is essentially the root of all evil. My approach isn't that extreme, but I do believe there is validity to the argument that there are times our body is more effective at healing itself than any pharmaceutical.

Before I get too far into this subject, I want to say that some medical conditions should be treated with medications. I also believe that nutritional therapy, particularly through a plant-based diet, is a strong, complementary therapy to any pharmacological protocol that a doctor orders. Pharmaceuticals, when necessary for the treatment of disease, work most effectively when the body is as nourished and balanced as possible. Changing your diet to include more plant-based foods can have a profound effect on the outcomes of medical treatment. If you have a serious health condition, please speak with a health care provider that can offer effective options for treatment.

With that disclaimer out of the way, I want to point out that the keyword in that last sentence is treatment. Your body needs a therapeutic approach that allows for treatment and full healing of disease and imbalances. Masking symptoms with medication might make you feel better, but it offers no curative effects.

Part of the reason I believe so strongly in your ability to treat disease without medication is that there are many diseases that we're living with today that have either minimal, experimental, or non-existent treatment options. Through my experience with clients, I have also witnessed first-hand how a dedicated approach to nourishing the body with a variety of plant-based foods has a therapeutic and restorative, healing effect. This is more than a fluffy theory based on anecdotal evidence. Science has been backing this for a long time.

Let's take autoimmune disorders for instance. Autoimmune conditions like MS or Crohn's disease have no known cure. With MS, the goal is to manage and slow the progression of symptoms, and medications that have made it onto the market are not curative. Instead they aim to slow symptoms, possibly by masking them, but the trade-off is a laundry list of side effects that some would consider worse than the disease itself. Other treatment options for MS are largely experimental, with unproven benefits. Crohn's disease is much the same, in that even surgery doesn't completely eliminate the disease. Medications are used to suppress the immune system and reduce inflammation but still, neither of these options treat the root cause of the disease – which is still unknown.

If you are already taking medication for a chronic health condition, such as an autoimmune disorder, do I want you to just stop taking your medication and eat a ton of vegetables instead? No, that would be reckless and possibly dangerous to your health. What I am presenting here is that with a dedicated approach to dietary changes, you may be able to reduce or eliminate medications used to treat your disease. If your disease is mild or in the early stages, you may be able to avoid pharmaceutical treatment altogether. A plant-based diet isn't a miracle cure for any disease, but it is a powerful healing tool that shouldn't be discounted.

To illustrate and back up my point, a study was conducted on patients with early-stage MS. The results revealed that a diet low in saturated fats that also restricted meat and dairy products is one of the most effective means of slowing the progression of MS. Personally, I think the numbers of this study are astounding. It found that 95% - meaning nearly all the participants – with early-stage MS were free of disease progression thirty or more years after adopting the dietary changes (Greger, 2013). This is incredible. We're talking about three decades or more of less suffering, less pain, and less disease – all because a choice was made to consume more plant-based foods in place of meat and dairy.

Another case study looked at the effects of adopting a plant-based diet to treat health conditions such as hypertension, diabetes, and heart disease (Tuso, Ismail, Ha, & Bartolotto, 2013). The results were overwhelmingly positive, with reports of patients being able to completely wean from their pharmaceutical treatments. The report also advocated that physicians encourage their patients to adopt plant-based diets. Additionally, it suggested that physicians move away from terms like vegan and vegetarian due to both their stigma and poorly defined nutritional concepts, in favor of the term plant-based, or simply encourage their patients to eat healthily and provide dietary guidelines that include abundant amounts of plant-based foods.

There is no shortage of anecdotal evidence to back up this study. Grammy award-winning singer Toni Braxton made headlines not that long ago when she disclosed that she had adopted a plant-based diet to manage and treat the symptoms of Lupus, which is another type of autoimmune disorder. I could go on here, but the point is you don't have to look too hard to find a story about how someone changed their life and healed their body by adopting a plant-based diet.

In an ideal world, you would be reading this book at the earliest onset of disease, or even before it has manifested in your body. The sooner you adopt a plant-based diet to treat hormonal and autoimmune dysfunction, the better. That said, even severe or late-stage autoimmune disorders show dramatic improvement when adopting a largely plant-based diet. Once the inflammation begins to subside, once food nourishes your body, as opposed to fighting against it, you begin to heal. It's never too late, or too early, to make these changes to rebuild and protect your health.

With or without medications, with or without the goal of weaning yourself from prescription pharmaceuticals, a plant-based diet can improve your health, heal your body, and potentially cure disease. Are you ready to embrace your own power over your health? I can't wait to see what the future holds for you.

CHAPTER SUMMARY

In this chapter, we discussed how to adopt a plant-based approach to eating that is sustainable for you. The goal is to make lifelong changes that will support your hormonal and autoimmune health through adopting a more plant-focused diet. Specifically, we've discussed:

- Making any type of dietary change to improve your health is a major change that requires commitment
- Remember that short-term results lead to successful long-term progress
- Take advantage of all the delicious sources of plant-based proteins to keep you satiated
- Through a plant-based approach to eating, many people can treat their chronic conditions without pharmaceuticals.

With everything you've learned, you're ready to take the first steps toward reclaiming your health by balancing hormones, regulating your endocrine function, and soothing the inflammation that is so prominent in every autoimmune disorder. It's in your hands now, and I have all the confidence in the world that you can do this.

7 DAY PLANT BASED MEAL PLAN WITH 21 RECIPES

To gain access to this chapter as a beautiful and colorful designed PDF where you will find all the recipes with colored images, then scan the QR code or use the link below. I hope you enjoy this delicious and tasteful add on.

SCAN ME

https://www.pureture.com/7-day-plant-based-meal-plan-w-21-recipes/

BREAKFAST: APPLE-LEMON BREAKFAST BOWL

This fresh apple-lemon breakfast bowl is beautifully flavored with dates, cinnamon, and walnuts. This breakfast is also deliciously filling and very nutritious.

INGREDIENTS:

- 4 to 5 medium apples, any variety
- 5 to 6 dates, pitted
- Juice of 1 lemon (about 3 tablespoons)
- 2 tablespoons of walnuts (about 6 walnut halves)
- ¼ teaspoon of ground cinnamon

INSTRUCTIONS:

1. Core the apples and cut into large pieces.
2. Place dates, half of the lemon juice, walnuts, cinnamon, and three quarters of the apple in the bowl of a food processor. Puree until finely ground, scraping down the sides of the bowl as needed.
3. Add the remainder of the apples and lemon juice and pulse until the apples are shredded and the date mixture is evenly distributed.

LUNCH: SPICY BUFFALO CHICKPEA WRAPS

I hope you'll love these wraps! They're:

- Savory
- Spicy
- Hearty
- Crunchy from the vegetables
- Tender from the chickpeas
- Quick
- Protein & fiber-filled
- Delicious

INGREDIENTS:

DRESSING + SALAD

- ⅓ cup of hummus (or store-bought)
- 1½ - 2 Tbsp of maple syrup (plus more to taste)
- 1 small lemon, juiced (1 small lemon yields ~2 Tbsp or 30 ml)
- 1-2 Tbsp of hot water (to thin)
- 1 head of romaine lettuce (or sub 1 bundle kale per 1 head romaine // cleaned, large stems removed, roughly chopped)

BUFFALO CHICKPEAS

- 1 15-ounce of can chickpeas (rinsed, drained and dried // ~ 1 ¼ cups per can when drained)
- 1 Tbsp of coconut oil (or sub grape seed or olive oil)
- 4 Tbsp of hot sauce (I used Louisiana's Pure Crystal Hot Sauce)
- ¼ tsp of garlic powder (or sub 1 minced garlic clove per ¼ tsp powder)
- 1 pinch of sea salt

FOR SERVING AND TOPPINGS

- 3-4 vegan-friendly flour tortillas, pita, or flatbread
- ¼ cup of red onion, diced (optional)
- ¼ cup of baby tomato, diced (optional)
- ¼ of a ripe avocado, thinly sliced (optional)

INSTRUCTIONS:

1. Make dressing by adding hummus, maple syrup, and lemon juice to a mixing bowl and whisking to combine. Add hot water until thick but pourable.
2. Taste and adjust flavor as needed, then add romaine lettuce or kale, and toss. Set aside.
3. To make chickpeas, add drained, dried chickpeas to a separate mixing bowl. Add coconut oil, 3 Tbsp hot

sauce, garlic powder, and a pinch of salt - toss to combine/coat.

4. Heat a metal or cast-iron skillet over medium heat. Once hot, add chickpeas and sauté for 3-5 minutes, mashing a few chickpeas gently with a spoon to create texture.

5. Once chickpeas are hot and slightly dried out, remove from heat and add remaining 1 Tbsp of hot sauce. Stir to combine. Set aside.

6. To assemble, top each wrap with a generous portion of the dressed romaine salad, and top with ¼ cup of buffalo chickpeas and a sprinkle of diced tomatoes, avocado, and/or onion (optional).

7. Serve immediately. Store leftovers separately in the refrigerator up to 3 days, though best when fresh. You can enjoy the buffalo chickpeas cold, room temperature or heated up.

DINNER: ROASTED CAULIFLOWER AND QUINOA CASSEROLE

This easy, cozy casserole melds tender quinoa with roasted cauliflower, green peas, and a zesty marinara sauce.

INGREDIENTS:

- 2 cups of dry quinoa
- 3½ cups of vegetable broth, divided

- ½ of a medium onion, cut into ¼-inch dice (1 cup)
- 6 cloves of garlic, minced
- 1 tablespoon of Italian seasoning
- 1 medium head of cauliflower, cut into 1-inch florets (about 6 cups)
- 1 tablespoon of white wine vinegar
- Sea salt and freshly ground black pepper
- 3 cups store-bought marinara sauce
- 1 cup of frozen green peas, thawed

INSTRUCTIONS:

1. In a large saucepan, combine quinoa and 3 cups of broth. Bring to a boil; then reduce heat to low and cover pan. Simmer for 20 minutes. Remove from heat and let it stand for 10 minutes. Drain off any excess water if needed.

2. In a skillet, combine onion, garlic, Italian seasoning, and ¼ cup broth; cook over medium for 10 minutes or until onion is tender, adding more broth, 1 to 2 tablespoons at a time, as needed to prevent sticking. Add cauliflower to skillet and cook 10 to 15 minutes more, or until cauliflower is starting to get tender. Do not overcook. Add vinegar and season with salt and pepper.

3. Preheat oven to 350°F. Fluff quinoa with a fork; then spread it in an even layer on the bottom of a large

casserole dish. Cover quinoa with an even layer of marinara sauce, followed by cauliflower and green peas on top. Bake uncovered 20 to 25 minutes until there is browning on the cauliflower. Serve warm.

BREAKFAST: CAULIFLOWER BREAKFAST SCRAMBLE

There are many very good recipes for scrambles, but most call for tofu. In this recipe, cauliflower takes the place of the tofu—with delicious results.

INGREDIENTS:

- 1 red onion, peeled and cut into ½-inch dice
- 1 red bell pepper, seeded and cut into ½-inch dice
- 1 green bell pepper, seeded and cut into ½-inch dice
- 2 cups of sliced mushrooms (from about 8 ounces whole mushrooms)
- 1 large head of cauliflower, cut into florets, or 2 (19-ounce) cans ackee, drained and gently rinsed
- Sea salt
- ½ teaspoon of freshly ground black pepper
- 1½ teaspoons of turmeric
- ¼ teaspoon of cayenne pepper, or to taste
- 3 cloves of garlic, peeled and minced
- 1 to 2 tablespoons of low-sodium soy sauce
- ¼ cup of nutritional yeast (optional)

INSTRUCTIONS:

1. Place the onion, red and green peppers, and mushrooms in a medium skillet or saucepan and sauté over medium-high heat for 7 to 8 minutes, or until the onion is translucent. Add 1 to 2 tablespoons of water at a time to keep the vegetables from sticking to the pan.
2. Add the cauliflower and cook for 5 to 6 minutes, or until the florets are tender.
3. Add the salt to taste, pepper, turmeric, cayenne, garlic, soy sauce, and nutritional yeast (if using) to the pan, and cook for 5 minutes more, or until hot and fragrant.

LUNCH: 5 MINUTE VEGGIE COCONUT WRAPS

Not only are they easy to make, requiring just *8 ingredients* and *5 minutes* to prepare, they are the ideal easy lunch or snack!

These are:

- Crunchy
- Flavor-packed
- Loaded with vegetables
- Fiber & Protein-rich
- Quick & easy
- Ridiculously delicious

INGREDIENTS:

- 5 Coconut Wraps (I love the Nuco Brand in turmeric flavor)
- ⅔ cup of hummus
- 7 ½ tbsp of green curry paste
- 1 red bell pepper - thinly sliced
- 1 cup of fresh cilantro (approximately 1 large bundle)
- 1 ½ cups of shredded carrots
- 1 ripe avocado - sliced
- 2 ½ cups of kale - chopped

INSTRUCTIONS:

1. Lay a single coconut wrap on a clean surface or cutting board. Add 2 Tbsp (~32 g) hummus and 1 ½ Tbsp curry paste (~22 g) and spread on the end of the wrap closest to you.
2. Add bell pepper, carrots, avocado, kale, and cilantro and roll tightly away from you. Place the seam side down on a serving platter. Repeat until you have 5 coconut wraps (or as many as you desire).
3. Best served fresh. Can store leftovers covered in the refrigerator up to 1 day.

DINNER: WHITE BEAN FETTUCCINE ALFREDO WITH PEAS AND SUN-DRIED TOMATOES

Fettuccine Alfredo has never been the healthiest pasta choice until now. In this version, a blended white bean sauce is used instead of cream, dried tomatoes take the place of bacon, and fresh sugar snap peas add more of a crunch and flavor than petite green peas.

INGREDIENTS:

- 8 oz. of dry whole wheat fettuccine
- 8 oz. of sugar snap peas, halved
- 1 15-oz. can of cannellini beans, rinsed and drained (1½ cups)
- 2 cloves of garlic
- 2 tablespoons of nutritional yeast
- 2 tablespoons of almond butter
- ⅓ cup of ready-to-eat sun-dried tomatoes, thinly sliced
- Sea salt and freshly ground black pepper to taste

INSTRUCTIONS:

1. Cook fettuccine according to package directions for al dente, adding peas the last 3 minutes of cooking. Drain, reserving ¾ cup cooking liquid.
2. Meanwhile, in a food processor, combine beans, garlic,

nutritional yeast, and almond butter. Process until
smooth. Add the reserved cooking liquid; process until
smooth.

3. Return pasta and peas to the pot. Stir in bean sauce and
tomatoes. Season with salt and pepper.

BREAKFAST: HEALTHY OATMEAL WITH FRUIT AND NUTS

Oatmeal is one of my favorite breakfast foods. It is quick to
prepare and easily adaptable to my ever-changing moods—some
days I want it with fruit, some days I want it plain, and sometimes I want a little of everything in it (that's when I include all
the optional ingredients listed here!). This basic recipe is all you
need to get started … add as much or as little of the extras as you
like.

INGREDIENTS:

- ¾ cup of rolled oats
- ¼ teaspoon of ground cinnamon
- Pinch of sea salt
- ¼ cup of fresh berries (optional)
- ½ of a ripe banana, sliced (optional)
- 2 tablespoons of chopped nuts, such as walnuts,
  pecans, or cashews (optional)
- 2 tablespoons of dried fruit, such as raisins,
  cranberries, chopped apples, chopped

- Apricots (optional)
- Maple syrup (optional)

INSTRUCTIONS:

1. Combine the oats and 1½ cups water in a small saucepan. Bring to a boil over high heat. Reduce the heat to medium-low and cook until the water has been absorbed, about 5 minutes.
2. Stir in the cinnamon and salt. Top with the berries, banana, nuts, and/or dried fruit, as you like. If desired, pour a little maple syrup on top. Serve hot.

LUNCH: ABUNDANCE KALE SALAD WITH SAVORY TAHINI DRESSING

An abundant kale salad with roasted sweet potato, zucchini, avocado, sprouts, crispy chickpeas, and kimchi! Topped with a savory tahini dressing, this salad makes the perfect 30-minute meal or side.

INGREDIENTS:

ROASTED VEGETABLES

- 1 medium zucchini (sliced in ¼-inch rounds)
- 1 medium sweet potato (sliced in ¼-inch rounds)
- 1 cup of red cabbage (shredded)

- 1 tbsp of melted coconut oil or sub water)
- 1 pinch sea salt
- ½ tsp of DIY curry powder (or store-bought)

DRESSING

- ⅓ cup of tahini
- ½ tsp of garlic powder (plus more to taste)
- 1 tbsp of coconut aminos (plus more to taste or sub tamari or soy sauce)
- 1 pinch of sea salt (omit if using tamari or soy sauce, as the flavor is more intense)
- 1 large clove of garlic (minced)
- ¼ cup of water (to thin)

SALAD

- 6 cups of mixed greens (kale, romaine, mixed greens, etc.)
- 4 small radishes (thinly sliced)
- 3 tbsp of hemp seeds
- 1 ripe avocado (cubed)
- 2 tbsp of lemon juice or apple cider vinegar

TOPPINGS optional / choose your favorites

- 1 batch of crispy baked chickpeas

- 2 cups of cooked quinoa
- DIY Kimchi (or store-bought)

INSTRUCTIONS:

1. If serving with quinoa or crispy chickpeas, prepare at this time. Otherwise, proceed to step 2.

2. Preheat the oven to 375 degrees F (190 C) and arrange zucchini, cabbage, and sweet potatoes on a baking sheet (one or more as needed). Drizzle with coconut oil (or sub oil-free options), sea salt, and curry powder and toss to combine. Roast for 20 minutes or until tender and slightly golden brown.

3. In the meantime, prepare dressing by adding tahini, garlic powder, coconut aminos, sea salt, and garlic to a small mixing bowl and whisking to combine. Then add enough water to thin until pourable and whisk until smooth. Taste and adjust seasonings as needed, adding more garlic powder for garlic flavor, coconut aminos for depth of flavor, or salt for saltiness. Set aside.

4. Assemble salad by adding greens, radishes, hemp seeds, and avocado to a large mixing bowl. Add the lemon juice (or apple cider vinegar) and gently toss to combine.

5. Add roasted vegetables and any other desired toppings (quinoa, chickpeas, etc.) and serve with dressing.

6. Best when fresh, though leftovers keep well stored in

the refrigerator up to 3 days. Dressing stored separately will keep for 7 days. Chickpeas should be stored separately at room temperature to maintain crispiness.

DINNER: LEMON BROCCOLI ROTINI

Enjoy the classic combination of broccoli, lemon, and tarragon in this creamy pasta dish. For the best presentation, use the same half of the lemon for the zest and juice, reserving the other half to cut into wedges for serving.

INGREDIENTS:

- 3 cups of sliced cremini mushrooms (8 oz.)
- 1 medium onion, chopped (1 cup)
- 4 cloves of garlic, minced
- 4 cups of dried whole wheat rotini pasta (12 oz.)
- 2 cups of low-sodium vegetable broth
- 2 cups of unsweetened, unflavored plant-based milk
- 1 lemon
- 1 16-oz. package frozen of broccoli florets (or 6 cups fresh)
- ½ cup of chopped roasted red bell peppers
- 1 teaspoon of chopped fresh tarragon
- Sea salt and freshly ground black pepper to taste

INSTRUCTIONS:

n a large saucepan cook mushrooms, onion, and garlic over medium 2 to 3 minutes, stirring occasionally and adding water, 1 to 2 Tbsp. at a time, as needed to prevent sticking. Stir in rotini, vegetable broth, and milk. Bring to boiling; reduce heat. Cover and simmer for 5 to 7 minutes or until pasta is nearly tender.

2. Remove 1 tsp. zest from lemon and stir into a saucepan with pasta. Stir in broccoli, red peppers, and tarragon. Cook for about 5 minutes or until broccoli and pasta are tender. Stir in 1 Tbsp. of juice from lemon. Season with salt and black pepper. If desired, sprinkle with additional lemon zest and serve with lemon wedges.

BREAKFAST: CHICKPEA OMELET

This wonderful egg-free omelet is easy to make and is delicious for breakfast, lunch, or dinner.

INGREDIENTS:

- 1 cup of chickpea flour
- ½ teaspoon of onion powder
- ½ teaspoon of garlic powder
- ¼ teaspoon of white pepper
- ¼ teaspoon of black pepper
- ⅓ cup of nutritional yeast
- ½ teaspoon of baking soda
- 3 green onions (white and green parts), chopped

- 4 ounces of sautéed mushrooms (optional)

INSTRUCTIONS:

1. Combine the chickpea flour, onion powder, garlic powder, white pepper, black pepper, nutritional yeast, and baking soda in a small bowl. Add 1 cup of water and stir until the batter is smooth.
2. Heat a frying pan over medium heat. Pour the batter into the pan, as if making pancakes. Sprinkle 1 to 2 tablespoons of the green onions and mushrooms into the batter for each omelet as it cooks. Flip the omelet. When the underside is browned, flip the omelet again, and cook the other side for a minute.
3. Serve your amazing Chickpea Omelet topped with tomatoes, spinach, salsa, hot sauce, or whatever heart-safe, plant-perfect fixings you like.

LUNCH: ROASTED RAINBOW VEGETABLE BOWL

This is a healthy, easy, and delicious roasted vegetable bowl with tahini dressing and hemp seeds! The perfect 30-minute plant-based meal for any time of the day!

INGREDIENTS:

VEGETABLES

- 3-4 medium red or yellow baby potatoes (sliced into ¼ -inch rounds)
- ½ of a large sweet potato (skin on // sliced into ¼ -inch rounds)
- 2 large carrots (halved and thinly sliced)
- 1 medium beet (sliced into ⅛ -inch rounds)
- 4 medium radishes (halved, or quartered if large)
- 2 tbsp of avocado oil or melted coconut oil
- 1 tsp of curry powder
- ½ tsp of sea salt (divided)
- 1 cup of cabbage (thinly sliced)
- 1 medium red pepper (thinly sliced)
- 1 cup of broccolini (roughly chopped)
- 2 cups of chopped collard greens or kale (organic when possible)

TOPPINGS

- 1 medium lemon (juiced or 3 Tbsp store bought lemon juice)
- 2 tbsp of tahini (divided)
- 2 tbsp of hemp seeds (divided)
- ½ of a medium avocado (divided // optional)

INSTRUCTIONS:

1. Preheat the oven to 400 degrees F (204 C) and line two baking sheets with parchment paper (or more baking sheets if increasing batch size).
2. To one baking sheet, add the potatoes, sweet potatoes, carrots, beets, and radishes and drizzle with half of the oil (or water), curry powder, and sea salt Toss to combine. Bake for 20-25 minutes or until golden brown and tender.
3. To the second baking sheet, add the cabbage, bell pepper, and broccolini. Drizzle with the remaining half of the oil (or water), curry powder, and sea salt. Toss to combine.
4. When the potatoes/carrots hit the 10-minute mark, add the second pan to the oven and bake for a total of 15-20 minutes. In the last 5 minutes of baking, add the collard greens or kale to either pan and roast until tender and bright green.
5. To serve, divide vegetables between serving plates and garnish with avocado (optional) and season with lemon juice, tahini, hemp seeds, and another pinch of sea salt (optional). You could also garnish with any fresh herbs you have!
6. Best when fresh. Store leftovers covered in the refrigerator for 3-4 days. Reheat in a 350-degree F (176

C) oven or on the stovetop over medium heat until hot.

DINNER: GARLICKY BOK CHOY NOODLE SOUP

The vegetables in this colorful noodle soup are just barely cooked, so they stay crisp in texture and bright in color. Baby bok choy, harvested when it's about 6 inches long, is milder and more tender than mature bok choy.

INGREDIENTS:

- 4 cups of no-salt-added vegetable broth
- 4 cloves of garlic, minced
- 1 tablespoon of minced fresh ginger
- 2 teaspoons of reduced-sodium soy sauce
- 6 ounces of dried brown rice pad Thai noodles
- 12 baby carrots with green tops, halved lengthwise, or 2 cups bias-sliced carrots
- 3 ounces of extra-firm light silken-style tofu, cut into ¼-inch cubes
- 2 heads of baby bok choy, halved lengthwise
- 12 thin spears of asparagus, trimmed
- 1 cup of fresh shiitake mushrooms, stems removed, or oyster mushrooms, sliced
- 4 scallions (green onions), green tops trimmed and cut in half lengthwise

- 1 lime, cut into wedges

INSTRUCTIONS:

1. In a 5- to 6-qt. pot, combine 4 cups of water, the broth, garlic, ginger, and soy sauce. Bring to boiling; reduce heat. Cover and simmer for 10 minutes to allow flavors to meld.
2. Add noodles, carrots, and tofu. Simmer, uncovered, 8 minutes, stirring occasionally. Add bok choy, asparagus, mushrooms, and scallions. Simmer, uncovered, 1 minute more. Serve in shallow bowls with lime wedges.

BREAKFAST: CHOCOLATE CHIP COCONUT PANCAKES

These pancakes are so simple and delicious, and they're just as good for dessert as they are for breakfast! Plus, they freeze really well, so you can make an extra batch and freeze them. Use a large griddle so that you can cook three or four at a time.

INGREDIENTS:

- 1 tablespoon of flaxseed meal
- 1¼ cups of buckwheat flour
- ¼ cup of old-fashioned rolled oats
- 2 tablespoons of unsweetened coconut flakes

- 1 tablespoon of baking powder
- Pinch of sea salt
- 1 cup of unsweetened, unflavored plant milk
- ½ cup of unsweetened applesauce
- ¼ cup of pure maple syrup
- 1 teaspoon of pure vanilla extract
- ⅓ cup of grain-sweetened, vegan mini chocolate chips
- Sliced bananas, for serving

INSTRUCTIONS:

1. Place the flaxseed meal in a small saucepan with ½ cup water. Cook over medium heat until the mixture gets a little sticky and appears stringy when it drips off a spoon, 3 to 4 minutes. Immediately strain the mixture into a glass measuring cup and set aside. Discard the seeds.

2. In a large bowl, whisk together the buckwheat flour, oats, coconut flakes, baking powder, and salt.

3. In a medium bowl, whisk together the milk, applesauce, maple syrup, vanilla, and 2 tablespoons of the reserved flax water.

4. Add the liquid mixture to the dry mix and stir together to blend; the batter will be thick. Stir in the chocolate chips.

5. Heat a nonstick griddle over medium-low heat. Pour ⅓ cup batter for each pancake onto the griddle and

spread gently. Cook for 6 to 8 minutes, until the pancakes look slightly dry on top, are lightly browned on the bottom, and release easily from the pan. Flip and cook for about 5 minutes on the other side.

6. Repeat for the remaining batter, wiping off the griddle between batches. Serve hot with sliced bananas.

Storage: Place cooked pancakes in an airtight container and refrigerate for up to 5 days or frozen for up to 1 month. Reheat pancakes in a 350°F oven for 15 minutes for refrigerated pancakes and 25 minutes if frozen.

LUNCH: VEGAN "BLT" SANDWICH

6-Ingredient vegan "BLT" sandwich made with vegan mayo and eggplant bacon! Crisp, smoky, flavorful, and so delicious.

INGREDIENTS:

- 2 slices of vegan bread
- 5-6 slices of eggplant bacon or ¼ cup of coconut bacon
- 2 tbsp of vegan mayo or hummus
- ¼ of a medium red or white onion (thinly sliced)
- ½ of a medium ripe tomato (thinly sliced)
- 2 leaves of green lettuce

INSTRUCTIONS:

1. Toast bread (optional). In the meantime, heat skillet over medium heat. Once hot, add eggplant bacon (if using coconut bacon, no need to heat) and cook for 1-2 minutes. Then flip and cook for another 1-2 minutes on the other side until warmed through. Remove from heat and set aside.

2. To assemble the sandwich, spread vegan mayo (or hummus) on the toasted bread slices. Then top one piece with Eggplant or Coconut Bacon, onion, tomato, and lettuce. Top with another piece of bread, slice (optional), and enjoy.

3. Could be made ahead of time (up to a few hours), but best when fresh.

DINNER: ROASTED VEGGIE FLATBREADS

Balsamic glaze is the perfect finishing touch for these flatbreads. When making it, watch carefully at the end so it doesn't scorch.

INGREDIENTS:

- Cornmeal, for dusting
- 1 recipe of homemade, oil free pizza dough
- 6 baby potatoes, quartered
- 8 brussels sprouts, quartered
- 1 medium carrot, coarsely chopped

- 1 medium shallot, coarsely chopped
- 1 tablespoon of red wine vinegar
- Sea salt and freshly ground black pepper, to taste
- ⅓ cup of balsamic vinegar
- 1 cup of no-salt-added canned cannellini beans, rinsed and drained
- 1 teaspoon of finely chopped fresh sage or ¼ tsp. dried sage, crushed
- 2 cups of fresh microgreen

INSTRUCTIONS:

1. Preheat the oven to 400°F. Lightly sprinkle a large baking sheet with cornmeal.
2. Divide dough into four portions. On a lightly floured surface, roll portions into 7- to 8-inch circles or 10×5-inch ovals. Transfer flatbreads to the prepared pan. Bake 10 to 13 minutes or until lightly browned and set (flatbreads may puff). Let cool.
3. Preheat the oven to 425°F. Line a 15×10-inch baking pan with foil. Arrange potatoes, Brussels sprouts, carrot, and shallot in a prepared baking pan. Sprinkle with red wine vinegar and season with salt and pepper. Roast about 20 minutes or until tender and lightly browned.
4. Meanwhile, for balsamic glaze, in a small saucepan bring balsamic vinegar to boiling; reduce heat.

Simmer, uncovered, about 6 minutes or until mixture has reduced to about 1 ½ Tbsp. and thickened to a syrup consistency.

5. In a bowl, mash beans with a fork and stir in sage and 2 tsp of water. Spread on flatbreads. Top with roasted vegetables. Remove foil from baking sheet; transfer flatbreads to baking sheet. Bake for 5 minutes to heat through.

6. Drizzle flatbreads with balsamic glaze and top with microgreens.

BREAKFAST: BLACK BEAN AND SWEET POTATO HASH

This black bean and sweet potato hash can be an ideal breakfast, a lunch, or a light dinner. It can be served simply as a side dish, spooned over brown rice or quinoa, wrapped in a whole-wheat tortilla, or made into soft tacos garnished with avocado, cilantro, and other favorite toppings. Make it in your Instant Pot or other pressure cooker, or do it the old-fashioned way, on the stovetop.

INGREDIENTS:

- 1 cup of chopped onion
- 1 to 2 cloves of garlic, minced
- 2 cups of peeled and chopped sweet potatoes (about 2 small or medium)

- 2 teaspoons of mild or hot chili powder
- ⅓ cup of low-sodium vegetable broth
- 1 cup of cooked black beans
- ¼ cup of chopped scallions
- Splash of hot sauce (optional)
- Chopped cilantro, for garnish

INSTRUCTIONS:

Stovetop Method

1. Place the onions in a nonstick skillet and sauté over medium heat, stirring occasionally, for 2 to 3 minutes. Add the garlic and stir.
2. Add the sweet potatoes and chili powder, and stir to coat the vegetables with the chili powder. Add broth and stir. Cook for about 12 minutes more, stirring occasionally, until the potatoes are cooked through. Add more liquid - 1 to 2 tablespoons at a time as needed, to keep the vegetables from sticking to the pan.
3. Add the black beans, scallions, and salt. Cook for 1 or 2 minutes more, until the beans are heated through.
4. Add the hot sauce (if using), and stir. Taste and adjust the seasonings. Top with chopped cilantro and serve.

Pressure Cooker Method

1. Heat a stovetop pressure cooker over medium heat or set an electric cooker to sauté. Add the onion and cook, stirring occasionally, for 2 to 3 minutes. Add the garlic and stir. Add the sweet potatoes and chili powder. Stir to coat the sweet potatoes with the chili powder. Add the broth and stir.

2. Lock the lid on the pressure cooker. Bring to high pressure for 3 minutes. Quick release the pressure. Remove the lid, tilting it away from you.

3. Add the black beans, scallions, and salt. Cook for 1 or 2 minutes more over medium heat, or lock on the lid for 3 minutes, until the beans are heated through.

4. Add the hot sauce (if using), and stir. Taste and adjust the seasonings. Top with chopped cilantro and serve.

LUNCH: CURRIED CAULIFLOWER, GRAPE & LENTIL SALAD

This crazy delicious kale salad is topped with red grapes, lentils, and curry roasted cauliflower. Served with a tahini-green curry paste dressing! Just 30 minutes required for this flavorful side or entrée.

INGREDIENTS:

CAULIFLOWER

- 1 head of cauliflower (divided into florets)
- 1 ½ tbsp of melted coconut oil (or water)
- 1 ½ tbsp of curry powder (or store-bought)
- ¼ tsp of sea salt

GREEN CURRY TAHINI DRESSING*

- 4 ½ tbsp of green curry paste (or store-bought, though fresh is best)
- 2 tbsp of tahini
- 2 tbsp of lemon juice
- 1 tbsp of maple syrup
- 1 pinch each of salt and black pepper
- Water to thin

SALAD

- 5-6 cups of mixed greens, kale, spinach (or other green of choice)
- 1 cup of cooked lentils (rinsed and drained)
- 1 cup of red or green grapes (halved)
- Fresh cilantro (optional)

INSTRUCTIONS:

1. Preheat the oven to 400 degrees F (204 C). Line a baking sheet (or more as needed) with parchment paper.
2. Add cauliflower to a mixing bowl and toss with coconut oil (or water), curry powder, and sea salt. Transfer to a baking sheet and roast cauliflower for 20-25 minutes or until golden brown and tender.
3. Prepare dressing by adding green curry paste, tahini, lemon juice, maple syrup, salt, and pepper to a mixing bowl and whisking to combine. If needed, thin with water until pourable.
4. Taste and adjust flavor as needed, adding more green curry paste for a stronger curry flavor, tahini for greater thickness, lemon juice for acidity, or maple syrup for sweetness.
5. Assemble salad by adding lettuce to a serving platter or bowl. Top with lentils, grapes, and cooked cauliflower and serve with dressing. Optional: garnish with fresh cilantro.
6. Best served fresh. Store leftovers in an airtight container for 3-4 days. Store dressing separately for up to 1 week.

DINNER: SPAGHETTI MARINARA WITH LENTIL BALLS

This whole-food vegan take on classic spaghetti and meatballs is as healthy as it is satisfying. The lentil "meatballs" take some time to make, but they're well worth the effort. They also freeze beautifully for up to a month: After baking, freeze them in an airtight container. Reheat in a 350°F oven 20 to 30 minutes.

INGREDIENTS:

- 1 cup of dry brown lentils, rinsed and drained
- 1 8-oz. package of button or cremini mushrooms, trimmed and chopped
- 1 onion, chopped (1 cup)
- 3 small cloves of garlic, minced
- ¼ cup of whole wheat or gluten-free flour
- 3 tablespoons of reduced-sodium tamari or soy sauce
- 2 tablespoons of no-salt-added tomato paste
- 1 tablespoon of nutritional yeast
- 1 teaspoon of dried oregano, crushed
- 1 teaspoon of onion powder
- Sea salt and freshly ground black pepper, to taste
- 1 lb. of dry gluten-free spaghetti
- 6 cups of oil-free marinara sauce
- 2 tablespoons of chopped fresh basil

INSTRUCTIONS:

1. In a large saucepan combine lentils and 1 cup of water. Bring to boiling; reduce heat. Cover and simmer for 15 minutes. Add mushrooms, onion, and garlic. Cover and cook about 15 minutes more or until lentils are tender. Uncover and cook until any remaining liquid has evaporated.

2. Stir in the next seven ingredients (through salt and pepper). Cook, uncovered, over low about 10 minutes or until liquid is absorbed and the pan is very dry, stirring occasionally. (Watch carefully so lentils do not scorch.) Spread mixture in a shallow baking pan; cool completely.

3. Preheat the oven to 250°F. Line a 15×10-inch baking pan with parchment paper. Scoop out 2 Tbsp. lentil mixture, shape into a ball, and place in the prepared pan. Repeat to make about 20 lentil balls. Bake for 45 minutes or until lightly browned and crisp.

4. Meanwhile, cook spaghetti according to package directions. In a saucepan heat marinara sauce. Drain spaghetti, return to pot, and toss with 3 cups of the warm marinara sauce.

5. To serve, top spaghetti with lentil balls and top with the remaining sauce. Sprinkle with basil.

BREAKFAST: EASY OVERNIGHT OATS WITH CHIA

To get through those busy weeks, try this easy and healthy breakfast that you can make the night before.

INGREDIENTS:

- ¾ cup of gluten-free rolled oats
- ¼ cup of plant-based milk
- ½ cup of water
- 1 heaping tablespoon of chia seeds
- ½ -1 tablespoon of maple syrup
- ¼ teaspoon of cinnamon
- Dash of vanilla bean powder or extract
- Fruit of choice

INSTRUCTIONS:

1. Place oats, liquid, chia seeds, maple syrup, cinnamon, and vanilla into a 16-ounce mason jar or container of choice. Mix well. Seal shut and place the jar in the refrigerator overnight.
2. In the morning, mix again and top with anything you'd like, such as fresh fruit, more chia seeds, or cacao nibs.

LUNCH: CHICKPEA QUINOA SALAD WITH ORANGE SOY & SESAME DRESSING

This hearty salad is absolutely loaded with good-for-you ingredients like chickpeas, quinoa, pumpkin seeds, sesame seeds, hemp seeds, kale, nutritional yeast, garlic, ginger, red and green bell peppers (just to name a few!) You can make this salad with quinoa or couscous. Quinoa has slightly more protein and quite a bit more fibre than couscous, but couscous is easier to prepare and cooks more quickly.

INGREDIENTS:

ORANGE SOY & SESAME DRESSING

- 1 navel orange, juiced
- 1 tbsp of sesame oil
- 1 tbsp of olive oil
- 1 tbsp of agave syrup
- 2 tbsp of soy sauce
- ½ tbsp of rice wine vinegar
- 1 ½ tbsp of nutritional yeast
- 2 cloves of garlic, minced
- ½" chunk of ginger, minced
- 1 tbsp of sesame seeds

CHICKPEA QUINOA SALAD

- 3 cups of quinoa, cooked (cook in broth for best flavour)
- 1 (540ml/19 fl. oz.) can of chickpeas, drained (approx. 2 cups cooked)
- ⅔ cup of chopped kale (stems removed, packed)
- ½ cup of chopped red and green bell pepper
- ¼ cup of chopped green onion
- ¼ cup of raw pumpkin seeds
- 2-4 tbsp of hemp hearts

INSTRUCTIONS:

ORANGE SOY & SESAME DRESSING

1. Combine all ingredients. Mix well and set aside.

CHICKPEA & QUINOA SALAD

1. If not already chilled, refrigerate cooked quinoa.
2. While the quinoa chills, combine kale with orange soy & sesame dressing. Set aside.
3. Combine room temperature (or cooler) quinoa, kale, dressing, and all remaining ingredients.
4. Refrigerate until chilled before serving.

DINNER: "STUFFINGED" SWEET POTATOES

These scrumptious stuffed sweet potatoes are worthy of center stage on a holiday table. Cremini mushrooms and chickpeas add lusciousness to a classic bread stuffing that is loaded with traditional flavor. This recipe requires only about 30 minutes of active prep time.

Tip: To dry bread cubes, spread them in a single layer in a baking pan. Let stand, uncovered, overnight. Or bake in a 300°F oven 10 to 15 minutes or until golden, stirring once or twice.

INGREDIENTS:

- 4 large sweet potatoes, scrubbed and patted dry (about 3 lb.)
- 1½ cups of chopped fresh cremini mushrooms (4 oz.)
- ½ cup of chopped onion
- 2 stalks celery, sliced (½ cup)
- 2 cloves of garlic, minced
- 2 15-oz. cans of no-salt-added chickpeas, rinsed and drained
- 2 cups of ½-inch whole wheat bread cubes, dried (see tip in intro)
- ½ cup of chopped fresh parsley
- 1½ teaspoon of poultry seasoning
- Sea salt and freshly ground black pepper, to taste
- ¼ to ⅓ cup of low-sodium vegetable broth

INSTRUCTIONS:

1. Preheat the oven to 400°F. Prick sweet potatoes all over with a fork. Place in a 3-qt. rectangular baking dish. Bake about 45 minutes or until just tender when pierced with a knife. Let stand until cool enough to handle.

2. Meanwhile, for stuffing, in a large nonstick skillet cook mushrooms, onion, celery, and garlic over medium 5 minutes, stirring occasionally and adding water, 1 to 2 Tbsp. at a time, as needed to prevent sticking.

3. In a food processor combine mushroom mixture and chickpeas; pulse until chopped. Transfer to a bowl. Add bread cubes, parsley, poultry seasoning, salt, and pepper. Drizzle with broth, tossing just until moistened.

4. Cut sweet potatoes in half lengthwise. Using a sharp knife, score around potato flesh, leaving a ¼-inch shell and being careful not to cut through skin. Score in a crisscross to make ½-inch cubes. Gently scoop cubes out with a spoon. If necessary, cut any large pieces in half to make smaller cubes. Add cubes to the stuffing mixture in a bowl; gently fold to combine.

5. Arrange potato skin shells in the baking dish. Spoon stuffing into shells. Bake, uncovered, about 20 minutes or until browned and heated through. To transport,

place the baking dish in an insulated carrier with a hot pack.

CHAPTER SUMMARY

In this last chapter, we provided you with a 7 day meal plan consisting of 3 meals per day. Specifically, we've shared:

- Breakfast recipes for 7 days;
- Lunch recipes for 7 days;
- Dinner recipes for 7 days;
- A total of 21 recipes to get you started in the right direction of adopting more of a plant-based lifestyle.

With everything you've learned, you're ready to take the first steps toward reclaiming your health by balancing hormones, regulating your endocrine function, and soothing the inflammation. Start with the given meal plan and play around along the way. I have all the confidence in the world that you can do this.

To gain access to this chapter as a beautiful and colorful designed PDF where you will find all the recipes with colored images, then scan the QR code or use the link below. I hope you enjoy this delicious and tasteful add on.

SCAN ME

https://www.pureture.com/7-day-plant-based-meal-plan-w-21-recipes/

CONCLUSION

I know that most of you haven't picked up this book because you're already in perfect health and just curious about the benefits of adopting a plant-based lifestyle. If that does describe you, I'm ecstatic that you've joined us but most of you reading this have either been diagnosed with hormonal or autoimmune dysfunction or strongly suspect that something is going haywire in your body.

My goal here has been to be your partner in restoring your health, and to provide you with a foundation of knowledge that covers the complete endocrine system, how it works, what sparks the manifestation of a disease, and how moving toward a plant-based diet can be therapeutic and healing. I know that each of you out there is coming from a different perspective, a different set of circumstances that makes your situation unique.

What I have aimed to provide is information and a path towards health that is uncomplicated, effective, and sustainable.

If there's one thing I want you to leave with, it's empowerment. I want you to feel empowered to take back control of your health. Empowered to seek options outside the standard medical conventions that have failed to treat the root of your disease. Empowered to make the best choices for your health. Empowered to be your own health advocate. Empowered to wake up in the morning and be free of pain and worry over your health. Empowered to live the healthy life you're deserving of.

I'm a huge proponent of the plant-based diet. I've witnessed firsthand with myself and my clients how eliminating disease and inflammation-causing foods can have a transformative effect. I'm also a realist. I know that a completely plant-based diet isn't going to fit in with everyone's lifestyle. This is why I've stressed that even just reducing, rather than eliminating, animal products is beneficial in the treatment of endocrine disorders and autoimmune disease in general. It's okay to go slow, as long as you're consistent in moving forward. This isn't an all or nothing scenario. This is about treating disease and restoring your health for life. It's a process, not a quick fix.

To summarize, here are a few of the main points that I hope you have gleaned from reading (and hopefully enjoying) this book.

- The endocrine system is a complex network of glands that regulate hormonal function
- The functions of the endocrine system affect every aspect of your health
- Endocrine dysfunction can manifest in many ways, often with unknown causes
- Autoimmune diseases are inflammatory conditions where the body's immune system attacks itself
- Modern pharmaceuticals overwhelmingly aim at relieving the symptoms of a disease, rather than the root cause of it
- Inflammation is a precursor to many of the chronic diseases we suffer from today
- How you nourish your body can have a profound effect on your health
- How plant-based diets nourish the body and also offer protection against oxidative stress and inflammation
- The anti-inflammatory effects of plant-based diets have been scientifically proven to relieve the inflammation associated with the development and progression of autoimmune disease
- In some cases, a plant-based diet has enabled people to completely wean from prescription pharmaceuticals
- Plant-based diets are associated with increased longevity
- Plant-based diets are associated with proper hormonal function

- Adopting a plant-based diet isn't an all or nothing venture
- Adopting a partially plant-based diet has been shown to have beneficial effects on health
- You're human. Give yourself grace, respect the process, and honor your body
- Adopting a plant-based lifestyle to heal your body is a lifelong process. There are no quick fixes or magic bullets to optimal health
- You are the only one that has the power to take control of your health. You need to make the commitment and follow the course
- You're not alone in this.

At this moment, you have the tools to make positive changes in your health. Now is the time to use them. Start today by making health goals for the future and taking those first steps toward healing. There's no better time to start than right now. Go out there and do it.

I hope you have not only enjoyed this book but that your health benefits from it as well. If you've found this book informative or have taken the plant-based plunge and changed your health, I would love to hear from you. Please leave a review, tell me what you think, and share the success of your journey with us.

I wish you success, health, and empowerment on this journey.

FINAL WORDS

If you enjoyed this book and are eager to get into a complete and very thorough process also known as a detoxification process then we want to recommend that you consider grabbing Pureture's detoxification book if you haven't already. This book is where we will walk you through step by step to cleanse, detox, and reset each organ in a safe, thorough and proper order. It is worth mentioning that the detox program is not only for plant-based eating, however, it does give plenty of options to choose from for people who choose to only eat plant-based. This program was created for people who do consume animal products and for people who don't.

Go ahead and look for the title:

"6 Optimal Steps for Detoxification & Reset; Ultimate Plan to Cleanse & Heal all Body Organs for Lasting Results"

This book has included a program that will absolutely change your life and get you on track for a lifelong lifestyle of healthy habits and staying cleansed. It has been geared to heal the gut and to also implement positive habits that will live with you forever.

MESSAGE FROM PURETURE WITH PURETURE WELLNESS

Thank you for giving yourself an opportunity to experience a change in your life. If any questions arise, or if you simply have a comment, please feel free to contact me through the website at https://www.pureture.com/. At Pureture Wellness, my team's mission is to expand the healing process that has changed our own lives so that we may impact as many as we can. At the link provided below, you may find some of my other work and related literature on the website as well.

I hope you have not only enjoyed this book but that your health benefits from it as well. If you've found this book informative or have taken the plant-based plunge and changed your health, I would love to hear from you. Please leave a review, tell me what you think, and share the success of your journey with us.

I wish you success, health, and empowerment on this journey.

Cheers to optimal health and wellness!

~Pureture, HHP

REFERENCES

Alwarith, J., Kahleova, H., Rembert, E., Yonas, W., Dort, S., Calcagno, M., . . . Barnard, N. (2019, September 10). Nutrition Interventions in Rheumatoid Arthritis: The Potential Use of Plant-Based Diets. A Review. Retrieved September 05, 2020, from https://www.ncbi.nlm.nih.gov/pmc/articles/PMC6746966/

Bolanowski, M., Halupczok, J., & Jawiarczyk-Przybyłowska, A. (2015, March 19). Pituitary Disorders and Osteoporosis. Retrieved September 05, 2020, from https://www.hindawi.com/journals/ije/2015/206853/

Centers for Disease Control and Prevention. (2017, July 18). New CDC report: More than 100 million Americans have diabetes or prediabetes. Retrieved September 05, 2020, from https://www.cdc.gov/media/releases/2017/p0718-diabetes-report.html

Centers for Disease Control and Prevention. (2019, October 23). Chronic Diseases in America. Retrieved September 05, 2020, from https://www.cdc.gov/chronicdisease/resources/infographic/chronic-diseases.htm

DeAngelis, T. (n.d.). The Two Faces of Oxytocin. Retrieved September 05, 2020, from https://www.apa.org/monitor/feb08/oxytocin

Delimaris, I. (2013, July 18). Adverse Effects Associated with Protein Intake above the Recommended Dietary Allowance for Adults. Retrieved September 05, 2020, from https://www.ncbi.nlm.nih.gov/pmc/articles/PMC4045293/

Duan, L., Rao, X., & Sigdel, K. (2019, February 28). Regulation of Inflammation in Autoimmune Disease. Retrieved September 05, 2020, from https://www.ncbi.nlm.nih.gov/pmc/articles/PMC6421792/

Elisei, R., & Alvarez, C. (n.d.). Thyroid. Retrieved September 05, 2020, from https://www.ese-hormones.org/focus-areas/thyroid/

GE;, S. (n.d.). Does low meat consumption increase life expectancy in humans? Retrieved September 05, 2020, from https://pubmed.ncbi.nlm.nih.gov/12936945/

Hayter, S., & Cook, M. (2012, February 23). Updated assessment of the prevalence, spectrum and case definition of autoimmune disease. Retrieved September 05, 2020, from https://www.sciencedirect.com/science/article/abs/pii/S1568997212000225?via=ihub

Houlihan, J., Lunder, S., & Jacob, A. (n.d.). Timeline: BPA from Invention to Phase-Out. Retrieved September 05, 2020, from https://www.ewg.org/research/timeline-bpa-invention-phase-out

Igbinedion, S., Ansari, J., Vasikaran, A., Gavins, F., Jordan, P., Boktor, M., & Alexander, J. (2017, October 28). Non-celiac gluten sensitivity: All wheat attack is not celiac. Retrieved September 05, 2020, from https://www.ncbi.nlm.nih.gov/pmc/articles/PMC5677194/

International Osteoporosis Foundation. (n.d.). Facts and Statistics. Retrieved September 05, 2020, from https://www.iofbonehealth.org/facts-statistics

National Cancer Institute. (n.d.). Medicinal Mushrooms (PDQ®)–Patient Version. Retrieved September 05, 2020, from https://www.cancer.gov/about-cancer/treatment/cam/patient/mushrooms-pdq

NCRAS. (n.d.). Thyroid cancer – trends by sex, age and histological type. Retrieved September 05, 2020, from http://www.ncin.org.uk/publications/

data_briefings/thyroid_cancer_trends_by_sex_age_and_histolog
ical_type

NIH. (n.d.). Lactose intolerance - Genetics Home Reference -
NIH. Retrieved September 05, 2020, from https://ghr.nlm.nih.
gov/condition/lactose-intolerance

Northwestern University. (2020, February 03). Eating red meat
and processed meat hikes heart disease and death risk, study
finds. Retrieved September 05, 2020, from https://www.
sciencedaily.com/releases/2020/02/200203114328.htm

Paturel, A. (n.d.). Is Dairy Arthritis Friendly. Retrieved
September 05, 2020, from https://www.arthritis.org/health-
wellness/healthy-living/nutrition/healthy-eating/dairy-and-
inflammation

Quagliani, D., & Felt-Gunderson, P. (2016, July 7). Closing
America's Fiber Intake Gap: Communication Strategies From a
Food and Fiber Summit. Retrieved September 05, 2020, from
https://www.ncbi.nlm.nih.gov/pmc/articles/PMC6124841/

Rasmussen, N., Rubin, K., Stougaard, M., Tjønneland, A.,
Stenager, E., Lund Hetland, M., . . . Andersen, V. (2019, March
30). Impact of red meat, processed meat and fibre intake on risk
of late-onset chronic inflammatory diseases: Prospective cohort
study on lifestyle factors using the Danish 'Diet, Cancer and
Health' cohort (PROCID-DCH): protocol. Retrieved September
05, 2020, from https://www.ncbi.nlm.nih.gov/pmc/
articles/PMC6475359/

Rosenfeld, D., & Tomiyama, A. (2019, September 23). Taste and health concerns trump anticipated stigma as barriers to vegetarianism. Retrieved September 05, 2020, from https://www.sciencedirect.com/science/article/pii/S0195666319310384

Tuso, P., Ismail, M., Ha, B., & Bartolotto, C. (2013). Nutritional update for physicians: Plant-based diets. Retrieved September 05, 2020, from https://www.ncbi.nlm.nih.gov/pmc/articles/PMC3662288/

U.S. Department of Health and Human Services. (n.d.). Chapter 2 Shifts Needed To Align With Healthy Eating Patterns. Retrieved September 05, 2020, from https://health.gov/our-work/food-nutrition/2015-2020-dietary-guidelines/guidelines/chapter-2/current-eating-patterns-in-the-united-states/

Wing, R., & Phelan, S. (2005, July 01). Long-term weight loss maintenance.Retrieved September 05, 2020, from https://academic.oup.com/ajcn/article/82/1/222S/4863393

Written By Michael Greger M.D. FACLM on May 21st, 2. (2013, May 21). Plant-Based Diets for Multiple Sclerosis. Retrieved September 05, 2020, from https://nutritionfacts.org/2013/05/21/plant-based-diets-for-multiple-sclerosis/

Zhang, Y., Li, S., Gan, R., Zhou, T., Xu, D., & Li, H. (2015, April 2). Impacts of gut bacteria on human health and diseases. Retrieved September 05, 2020, from https://www.ncbi.nlm.nih.gov/pmc/articles/PMC4425030/

To gain access to this chapter as a beautiful and colorful designed PDF where you will find all the recipes with colored images, then scan the QR code or use the link below. I hope you enjoy this delicious and tasteful add on.

SCAN ME

https://www.pureture.com/7-day-plant-based-meal-plan-w-21-recipes/

Printed in Great Britain
by Amazon